HOT TOPICS IN ECHOCARDIOGRAPHY

Edited by **Angelo Squeri**

Hot Topics in Echocardiography
http://dx.doi.org/10.5772/57354
Edited by Angelo Squeri

Contributors

Gheorghe Cerin, Ernesto Salcedo, Lucia Agoston-Coldea, Bruce Johnson, Ryotaro Wake

Published by InTech

Janeza Trdine 9, 51000 Rijeka, Croatia

Publishing Process Manager Sandra Bakic
Technical Editor InTech DTP team
Cover InTech Design team

Additional hard copies can be obtained from orders@intechopen.com

Hot Topics in Echocardiography, Edited by Angelo Squeri
p. cm.
ISBN 978-953-51-1204-4

For EU product safety concerns:
IN TECH d.o.o., Prolaz Marije Krucifikse Kozulić 3, 51000 Rijeka, Croatia,
info@intechopen.com or visit our website at intechopen.com.

Meet the editor

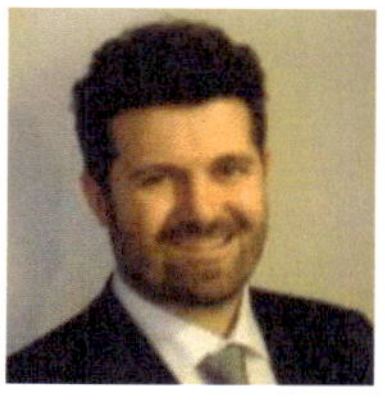

Angelo Squeri MD is a clinical cardiologist at Maria Cecilia Hospital, GVM Care & Research (Cotignola, Italy). He graduated in medicine in 2003 at the Università degli Studi di Parma where he also received his fellowship in Cardiology. He developed his interest in echocardiography especially in stress echocardiography with myocardial perfusion study, publishing several articles in the field of coronary artery disease. He also developed an expertise in valvular heart disease and three dimensional echocardiography, becoming lead of the TAVI and MitraClip imaging program at Maria Cecilia Hospital. He is a member of the European Association of Cardiovascular Imaging, European Working group on valvular heart disease and Associazione Nazionale dei Medici Cardiologi Ospedalieri. He has also been an invited speaker at a number of international meetings and serves as reviewer for several journals.

Contents

Preface

Echocardiography, despite the huge development of computed tomography and magnetic resonance imaging, is still the most used imaging technique for the evaluation of cardiac anatomy and function and today it plays an essential role in daily decision making.

Echocardiography offers a number of advantages over newer and more sophisticated technologies. First of all echocardiography offers a complete morphological and hemodynamic evaluation. Furthermore ultrasounds are radiation and contrast free, they are widely available, relatively cheap and they can be performed at the patient's bed, even to very critical ones.

Cardiologists face unique challenges interpreting echocardiographic imaging and trough the integration of these data with other clinical information.

Heart failure is becoming increasingly common and a major clinical and public health challenge. The prevalence of the disease is rising mainly because the population is getting older. More people survive myocardial infarction and some of them will develop heart failure. An increasing fraction, especially older, diabetic, hypertensive patients, and those with atrial fibrillation, exhibit heart failure with preserved systolic function. Echocardiography meets the growing need for non-invasive imaging in the expanding heart failure population because of its ability to provide accurate measures of ventricular function, filling pressure and to asses causes of structural heart disease. Echocardiography offers also prognostic information and can guide the therapy.

The echocardiographic technology and its applications have widely developed in the last years leading to a better diagnostic accuracy. On the other hand echocardiography specialists have new clinical questions to answer.

Since the introduction of percutaneous closure of patent foramen ovale, atrial and ventricular septal defects, echocardiography has become the imaging technique of choice in selection of patients and during the percutaneous procedure in the cath lab.

In the last years new structural heart interventions have become widely available such as, transcatheter aortic valve replacement, mitral valve repair, mitral valvuloplasty and left atrial appendage closure. These new percutaneous therapies need, in particular during the patients selection phase, a precise evaluation of cardiac dimensions and a complete understanding of the spatial relationships between cardiac structures. Echocardiography is of paramount importance both during the patient evaluation and guiding the procedure.

Three dimensional echocardiography, especially in the transesophageal approach, is a key technique for a precise localization and an easier definition of cardiac anatomy.

This book tries to give an in depth evaluation about the specific issues that a modern cardiovascular imaging specialist is asked to answer nowadays.

Dr. Angelo Squeri
Cardiology
Maria Cecilia Hospital, Cotignola (RA)
Italy

Chapter 1

Echocardiographic Evaluation of Left Ventricular Diastolic Function

Ryotaro Wake, Shota Fukuda, Hiroki Oe, Yukio Abe, Junichi Yoshikawa and Minoru Yoshiyama

Additional information is available at the end of the chapter

http://dx.doi.org/10.5772/55619

1. Introduction

The mortality, hospitalization, and prevalence rates of heart failure (HF) are increasing, in spite of decrease in coronary artery and cerebrovascular disease mortality.[1]

Approximately half of patients with a diagnosis of heart failure have a normal left ventricular (LV) ejection fraction (EF) without valve disease which is defined as diastolic heart failure (DHF), because it is attributed to LV diastolic dysfunction.[2] Studies examining prevalence of diastolic heart failure in hospitalized patients or in patients undergoing outpatient diagnostic screening and prospective community based studies have shown that the prevalence of diastolic heart failure approaches 50%.[3-5]

They tend to be older and female, and their condition is likely to be associated with hypertension, diabetes mellitus and ischemic heart disease. Many reports show that the mortality and morbidity of DHF is minimal differences from that of HF with a reduced EF. Moreover, although the mortality and morbidity have improved for patients with HF with a reduced EF, it has not changed for patients with DHF. So, the Evaluation of LV diastolic function is important.

LV diastolic function is related to myocardial relaxation and passive LV properties and is modulated myocardial tone. Myocardial relaxation is an active process, while stiffness is on the contrary a mechanical property of the myocardial wall.

Echocardiography is useful for the evaluation of LV diastolic function. The points of diastolic function to be estimated with echocardiography are propagation velocities, pulmonary vein Doppler, mitral inflow pattern and tissue Doppler imaging. We discuss the estimation of LV diastolic function with echocardiography.

2. The mechanism of DHF

Heart failure is a clinical syndrome characterized by symptoms and signs of increased tissue water and decreased tissue perfusion. Definition of the mechanisms that cause this clinical syndrome requires measurement of both systolic and diastolic function. When heart failure is accompanied by a predominant or isolated abnormality in diastolic function, this clinical syndrome is called diastolic heart failure. The pathophysiology is attributed to LV diastolic dysfunction, in which LV diastolic chamber size is normal or reduced despite elevated filling pressures resulting in decreased cardiac output. DHF occurs when the ventricular chamber is unable to accept an adequate volume of blood during diastole, because of a decrease in ventricular relaxation and/or an increase in ventricular stiffness,[2] and increased circulating blood volume is present. Hypertension, ischemia, aging and diabetes mellitus are the major risk factor of a decrease in ventricular relaxation and/or an increase in ventricular stiffness. Endocardial biopsies from HF patients without coronary artery disease (CAD) showed structural and functional differences in cardiomyocytes from patients with diastolic HF compared to cardiomyocytes from patients with abnormal systolic ejection fraction.[6] Myocytes from patients with diastolic HF had increased diameter and higher myofibrillar density and developed greater passive force and had greater calcium sensitivity. Myocardial collagen volume fraction was equally elevated.

Patients with DHF were shown to have similar pathophysiological characteristics, compared with HF patients with a reduced EF including reduced exercise capacity and impaired quality of life. DHF will be present in heart failure with preserved ejection fraction. When it is difficult with diagnosing HF, it is important to use echocardiography. [7,8]

2.1. The diagnosis of DHF

The diagnosis of heart failure with preserved left ventricular (LV) ejection fraction (HFpEF) requires the following conditions to be satisfied: (1) signs or symptoms of heart failure; (2) normal or mildly abnormal systolic LV function; (3) evidence of diastolic LV dysfunction. Normal or mildly abnormal systolic LV function implies both an LVEF > 50% and an LV end-diastolic volume index (LVEDVI) < 97 mL/m^2. Diagnostic evidence of diastolic LV dysfunction can be obtained invasively (LV end-diastolic pressure >16 mmHg or mean pulmonary capillary wedge pressure >12 mmHg) or non-invasively by tissue Doppler imaging (TDI) (E/E′ >15) with an echocardiography. If TDI yields an E/E′ ratio suggestive of diastolic LV dysfunction (8 < E/E′ < 15), additional non-invasive investigations are required for diagnostic evidence of diastolic LV dysfunction. These can consist of blood flow Doppler of mitral valve or pulmonary veins, echocardiographic measures of LV mass index or left atrial volume index, electrocardiographic evidence of atrial fibrillation, or plasma levels of natriuretic peptides. If plasma BNP is more than 200 pg/mL, diagnostic evidence of diastolic LV dysfunction also requires additional non-invasive investigations.

A similar strategy with focus on a high negative predictive value of successive investigations is proposed for the exclusion of HFpEF in patients with breathlessness and no signs of congestion. If a patient with breathlessness and no signs of fluid overload has a BNP of less

http://dx.doi.org/10.5772/55619

than 100 pg/mL, any form of heart failure is virtually ruled out because of the high negative predictive value of the natriuretic peptides, and pulmonary disease becomes the most likely cause of breathlessness. [9, 10]

As far as diastolic dysfunction, in decompensated patients with advanced systolic heart failure (LVEF≦30%, New York Heart Association class III to IV symptoms), tissue Doppler-derived with E/E′ ratio may not be as reliable in predicting intracardiac filling pressures, particularly in those with larger LV volumes, more impaired cardiac indices, and the presence of cardiac resynchronization therapy. [11]

2.2. Echocardiography in LV diastolic dysfunction

2.2.1. Doppler echocardiographic assessment of diastolic function and filling pressures

Comprehensive Doppler echocardiography is invaluable in the evaluation of HF patients. It is established that the mitral E wave velocity reflects the LA-LV pressure gradient during early diastole and is therefore affected by preload and alterations in LV relaxation. Assessment of diastolic function begins with the transmitral flow velocity profile. Decreases in the ratio of early to late diastolic filling (E/A), increases in the deceleration time, increases in the isovolumic relaxation time, or increases in tissue Doppler imagings (E/E′) indicate impaired relaxation. However, in the presence of impaired relaxation, increases in filling pressure progressively modify the transmitral gradient and mitral inflow pattern. A comprehensive Doppler assessment must be used to determine diastolic function from filling pressures and tissue Doppler imagings. [10] Patients studied at various times during their presentation will display a spectrum of filling patterns, including abnormal relaxation and psuedonormal or restrictive patterns. Such a spectrum has also been reported in patients with HF with a depressed EF and reflects the potent effect of filling pressures and blood pressure and their interaction with underlying diastolic dysfunction on the Doppler patterns. Thus, depending on their level of compensation and their filling pressures and whether they have exertional or rest symptoms, patients with HFpEF may display any of the filling patterns.[12]

2.2.2. Tissue Doppler imaging

Tissue Doppler imaging (TDI) is performed in the apical views to acquire mitral annular velocities with pulse wave. The sample volume should be positioned at 1 cm within the septal and lateral insertion sites of the mitral leaflets. It is recommended that spectral recordings be obtained at a sweep speed of 50 to 100 mm/s at end-expiration and that measurements should reflect the average of more than 3 consecutive cardiac cycles. Primary measurements include the systolic and early (e′) and late (a′) diastolic velocities. For the assessment of global LV diastolic function, it is recommended to acquire and measure tissue Doppler signals at least at the septal and lateral sides of the mitral annulus and their average. In patients with cardiac disease, e′ can be used to correct for the effect of LV relaxation on mitral E velocity, and the E/e′ ratio can be applied for the prediction of LV filling pressures. The E/e′ ratio is not accurate as an index of filling pressures in normal subjects or in patients with heavy annular calcification, mitral valve disease, and constrictive pericarditis.

Strain and strain rate can be derived from either tissue Doppler or speckle tracking 2-dimensional echocardiography. Using tissue Doppler, which is a form of pulsed Doppler, specific points within the myocardium can be identified. Tracking these Doppler points enables measurement of strain rate. Because Doppler is velocity or distance divided by time, the initial measurement is strain rate. Integrating the strain rate gives strain. The estimation of strain in the global left ventricular wall is called as global longitudinal strain (GLS).

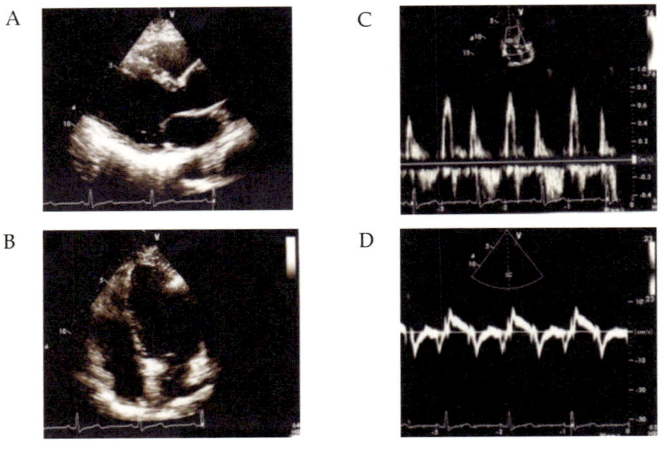

Figure 1. Normal pattern in LV inflow: Panel A shows long axis view. Panel B shows 4 chamber view. Panel C shows LV inflow. Panel D shows tissue Doppler imaging.

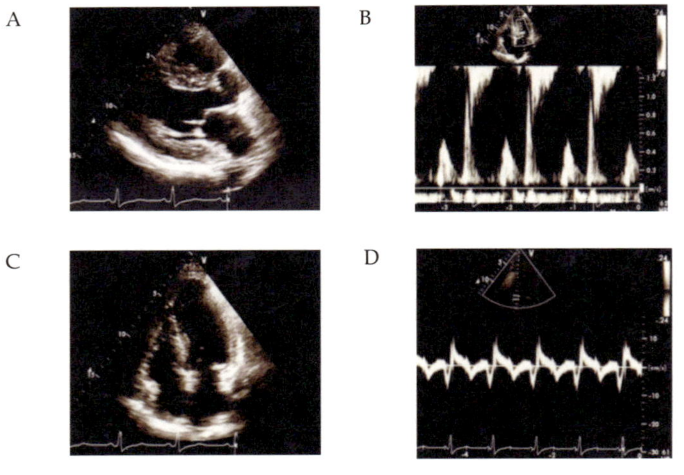

Figure 2. Abnormal relaxation pattern in LV inflow: Panel A shows long axis view. Panel B shows 4 chamber view. Panel C shows LV inflow. Panel D shows tissue Doppler imaging.

http://dx.doi.org/10.5772/55619

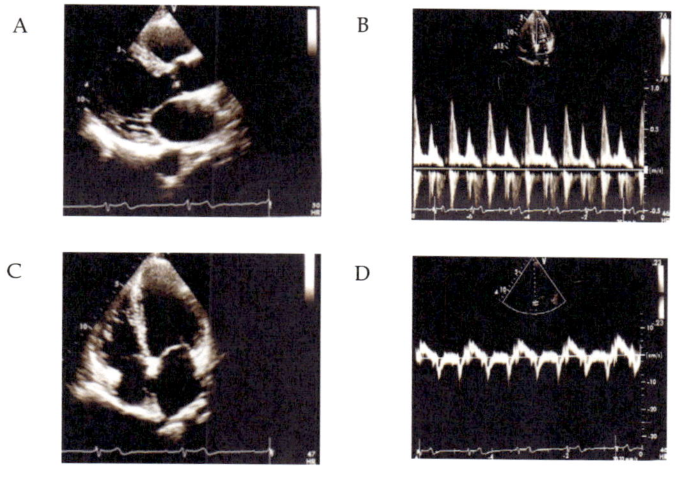

Figure 3. Pseudonormalized pattern in LV inflow: Panel A shows long axis view. Panel B shows 4 chamber view. Panel C shows LV inflow. Panel D shows tissue Doppler imaging.

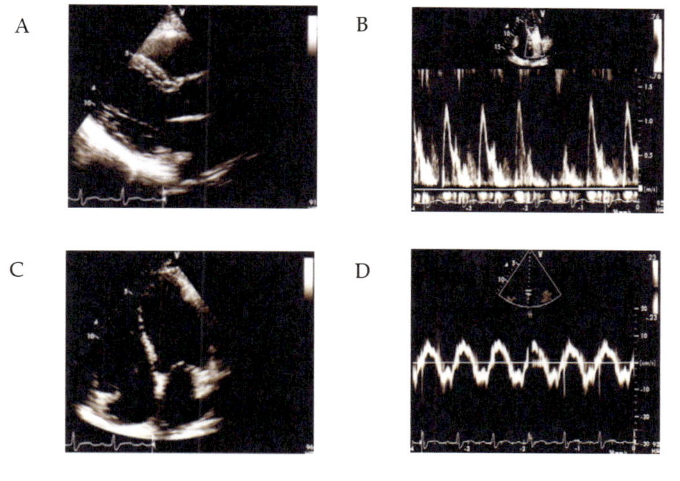

Figure 4. Restrictive pattern in LV inflow: Panel A shows long axis view. Panel B shows 4 chamber view. Panel C shows LV inflow. Panel D shows tissue Doppler imaging.

2.2.3. *Left ventricle in diastolic heart failure*

Most patients with HFpEF have normal chamber dimensions, although a small subset may have variable degrees of LV enlargement.

Although HF preserved EF has been thought to occur primarily patients with left ventricular hypertrophy (LVH), studies that have carefully quantified LV mass report that echocardiographic criteria for LVH are met in less than 50% of patients. [13-16]

2.2.4. Left atrium in diastolic heart failure

Increases in the left atrial dimension or volume are commonly present in patients with HF preserved EF. [17-19] The left atrium modulates ventricular filling through its reservoir, conduit, and pump functions. During ventricular systole and isovolumic relaxation, when the atrioventricular (AV) valves are closed, atrial chambers work as distensible reservoirs accommodating blood flow from the venous circulation. The atrium is also a pumping chamber, which contributes to maintaining adequate LV end-diastolic volume by actively emptying at end-diastole. Finally, the atrium behaves as a conduit that starts with AV valve opening and terminates before atrial contraction and can be defined as LV stroke volume minus the sum of LA passive and active emptying volumes.

The measurement of left atrial (LA) volume is highly feasible and reliable in most echocardiographic studies, with the most accurate measurements obtained using the apical 4-chamber and 2-chamber views. This assessment is clinically important, because there is a significant relation between LA remodeling and echocardiographic indices of diastolic function. In the previous observational studies, patients without baseline histories of atrial fibrillation and significant valvular heart disease have shown that more than 34 mL/m^2 LA volume index is an independent predictor of death, heart failure, atrial fibrillation, and ischemic stroke.

The dilated left atria may be seen in patients with bradycardia and 4-chamber enlargement, anemia and other high-output states, atrial flutter or fibrillation, and significant mitral valve disease, in the absence of diastolic dysfunction. Likewise, it is often present in elite athletes in the absence of cardiovascular disease. Therefore, it is important to consider LA volume measurements in conjunction with a patient's clinical status, other chambers' volumes, and Doppler parameters of LV relaxation.

2.2.5. Pulmonary hypertension in diastolic heart failure

Symptomatic patients with diastolic dysfunction usually have increased pulmonary artery (PA) pressures. [17,20] Therefore, in the absence of pulmonary disease, increased PA pressures may be used to infer the presence of elevated LV filling pressures. Indeed, a significant correlation was noted between PA systolic pressure and noninvasively derived LV filling pressures. The peak velocity of the tricuspid regurgitation (TR) jet by continuous-wave (CW) Doppler together with systolic right atrial (RA) pressure are used to derive PA systolic pressure. In patients with severe TR and low systolic right ventricular–RA pressure gradients, the accuracy of the PA systolic pressure calculation is dependent on the reliable estimation of systolic RA pressure. Likewise, the end-diastolic velocity of the pulmonary regurgitation (PR) jet can be applied to derive PA diastolic pressure. Both signals can be enhanced, if necessary, using agitated saline or intravenous contrast agents, with care to avoid overestimation caused by excessive noise in the signal. The estimation of RA pressure is needed for both calculations and can be derived using inferior vena caval diameter and its change with respiration, as well as the ratio of systolic to diastolic flow signals in the hepatic veins.

2.2.6. Pulmonary venous flow

Pulse wave (PW) Doppler of pulmonary venous flow is performed in the apical 4-chamber view and aids in the assessment of LV diastolic function. A 2-mm to 3-mm sample volume is placed more than 0.5 cm into the pulmonary vein for optimal recording of the spectral waveforms. Measurements include peak S and D velocities, the S/D ratio, systolic filling fraction, and peak Ar velocity in late diastole. Another measurement is the time difference between Ar duration and mitral A-wave duration (Ar - A). With increased LV end-diastolic pressure, Ar velocity and duration increase, as well as the Ar - A duration. In patients with depressed EFs, reduced systolic filling fractions (less than 40%) are related to decreased LA compliance and increased mean LA pressure. Atrial fibrillation results in a blunted S wave and absence of Ar velocity.

2.2.7. Other echocardiographic findings in diastolic heart failure

Regional wall motion abnormalities with preserved EF and right ventricular dilatation, either from ischemic disease or secondary to chronic pressure overload from chronic pulmonary venous hypertension, can also be present at echocardiography in patients with HFpEF. Additional negative findings at echocardiography include the absence of valvular disease, pericardial tamponade, pericardial constriction, the presence of congenital heart diseases such as atrial septal defect, other more extensive structural abnormalities are important enough to cause the HF symptoms.

3. Conclusions

HFpEF currently accounts for more than 50% of all heart failure patients. The updated strategies for the diagnosis and exclusion of HFpEF are useful not only for individual patient management but also for patient recruitment in future clinical trials exploring therapies for HFpEF. Echocardiography is useful for the diagnosis of HFpEF, noninvasively.

Author details

Ryotaro Wake*, Shota Fukuda, Hiroki Oe, Yukio Abe, Junichi Yoshikawa and Minoru Yoshiyama

*Address all correspondence to: wake123aha@yahoo.co.jp

Osaka City University Graduate School of Medicine, Japan

References

[1] Braunwald, E. (1997). Shattuck lecture--cardiovascular medicine at the turn of the millennium: triumphs, concerns, and opportunities. *N Engl J Med* 337 (19), 1360-1369

[2] Redfield, M. M. (2004). Understanding "diastolic" heart failure. *N Engl J Med* 350 (19), 1930-1931

[3] Aurigemma, G. P, et al. (2001). Predictive value of systolic and diastolic function for incident congestive heart failure in the elderly: the cardiovascular health study. *J Am Coll Cardiol* 37 (4), 1042-1048

[4] Gottdiener, J. S, et al. (2000). Predictors of congestive heart failure in the elderly: the Cardiovascular Health Study. *J Am Coll Cardiol* 35 (6), 1628-1637

[5] Kitzman, D. W, et al. (2001). Importance of heart failure with preserved systolic function in patients > or = 65 years of age. CHS Research Group. Cardiovascular Health Study. *Am J Cardiol* 87 (4), 413-419

[6] Van Heerebeek, L, et al. (2006). Myocardial structure and function differ in systolic and diastolic heart failure. *Circulation* 113 (16), 1966-1973

[7] Prasad, A, et al. (2005). Abnormalities of Doppler measures of diastolic function in the healthy elderly are not related to alterations of left atrial pressure. *Circulation* 111 (12), 1499-1503

[8] Zile, M. R, & Brutsaert, D. L. (2002). New concepts in diastolic dysfunction and diastolic heart failure: Part I: diagnosis, prognosis, and measurements of diastolic function. *Circulation* 105 (11), 1387-1393

[9] Paulus, W. J, et al. (2007). How to diagnose diastolic heart failure: a consensus statement on the diagnosis of heart failure with normal left ventricular ejection fraction by the Heart Failure and Echocardiography Associations of the European Society of Cardiology. *Eur Heart J* 28 (20), 2539-2550

[10] Redfield, M. M, et al. (2003). Burden of systolic and diastolic ventricular dysfunction in the community: appreciating the scope of the heart failure epidemic. *JAMA* 289 (2), 194-202

[11] Mullens, W, et al. (2009). Tissue Doppler imaging in the estimation of intracardiac filling pressure in decompensated patients with advanced systolic heart failure. *Circulation* 119 (1), 62-70

[12] Bursi, F, et al. (2006). Systolic and diastolic heart failure in the community. *JAMA* 296 (18), 2209-2216

[13] Chen, H. H, et al. (2002). Diastolic heart failure in the community: clinical profile, natural history, therapy, and impact of proposed diagnostic criteria. *J Card Fail* 8 (5), 279-287

[14] Kawaguchi, M, et al. (2003). Combined ventricular systolic and arterial stiffening in patients with heart failure and preserved ejection fraction: implications for systolic and diastolic reserve limitations. *Circulation* 107 (5), 714-720

[15] Kitzman, D. W, et al. (2002). Pathophysiological characterization of isolated diastolic heart failure in comparison to systolic heart failure. *JAMA* 288 (17), 2144-2150

[16] Zile, M. R, et al. (2004). Diastolic heart failure--abnormalities in active relaxation and passive stiffness of the left ventricle. *N Engl J Med* 350 (19), 1953-1959

[17] Lam, C. S, et al. (2009). Pulmonary hypertension in heart failure with preserved ejection fraction: a community-based study. *J Am Coll Cardiol* 53 (13), 1119-1126

[18] Lam, C. S, et al. (2007). Cardiac structure and ventricular-vascular function in persons with heart failure and preserved ejection fraction from Olmsted County, Minnesota. *Circulation* 115 (15), 1982-1990

[19] Melenovsky, V, et al. (2007). Cardiovascular features of heart failure with preserved ejection fraction versus nonfailing hypertensive left ventricular hypertrophy in the urban Baltimore community: the role of atrial remodeling/dysfunction. *J Am Coll Cardiol* 49 (2), 198-207

[20] Kjaergaard, J, et al. (2007). Prognostic importance of pulmonary hypertension in patients with heart failure. *Am J Cardiol* 99 (8), 1146-1150

Chapter 2

Right Chambers Quantification in Clinical Practice: Echocardiography Compared with Cardiac Magnetic Resonance Imaging

Lucia Agoston-Coldea and Silvia Lupu

Additional information is available at the end of the chapter

http://dx.doi.org/10.5772/55832

1. Introduction

The right ventricle (RV) has its own particular morphology and functions, which are different when compared to the left ventricle (LV). In clinical practice, the right heart chambers are often overlooked, as most physicians tend to focus more on LV and left atrium (LA) morphology and functions. However, cardiac pathology is often associated with right chambers impairment, which can occur as a primary pathophysiological response to elevated pressure in the pulmonary arterial circulation associated with primary pulmonary artery hypertension [1-2], in pulmonary diseases associated with pulmonary venous or arterial hypertension [3-4], pulmonary embolism [5], but also in congenital heart disease [6]. Most often, RV dysfunction is triggered by left chamber impairment [7-9].

Right cardiac imaging is quite challenging, as there are few validated and reproducible parameters that can be employed for an accurate right atrium (RA) and RV morphology and function assessment. However, some imaging techniques are available for this purpose. Nowadays, cardiac magnetic resonance imaging (MRI) is the golden standard for right chambers evaluation [10], due to its unlimited imaging planes, higher image resolution, and the ability to calculate volumes using three-dimensional (3D) measurements. Regrettably, this type of evaluation is not available in many centres and rather expensive, requiring high quality equipment and highly trained examiners.

Although cardiac MRI is the preferred method [11], echocardiography remains a valuable alternative, as it is widely available, non-invasive, and less expensive and can be performed in all patients oblivious of associated pathology or the presence of metallic devices such as pacemakers, implanted cardioverter defibrillators, cochlear implants or drug infusion pumps.

Some studies seem to suggest that the risk usually associated with cardiac MRI in patients with pace makers and defibrillators is overestimated and that examination using magnetic fields up to 1.5 Tesla can be safe [12-13]. However, performing such an examination is not without risk and should be attempted in selected patients, with several precautions including complete resuscitation facilities and in the presence of an electrophysiologist [14]. All in all, cardiac MRI requires many precautions, in such cases, whereas echocardiography is without risk and easier to perform. Despite its major advantages, echocardiography has its limitations, mainly due to the particular morphology of the RV. The thin, trabeculated right free wall and the anterior position in the chest render RV assessment difficult [15]. Moreover, endocardial border tracing is strenuous due to the presence of trabeculations, which can be a source of error when attempting to obtain precise dimension assessment. These downfalls are limited when real-time 3D echocardiography is used, although, for the time being, end-systolic and end-diastolic RV volumes seem to be underestimated when compared to cardiac MRI measurements [16]. Some studies have shown, however, that, in spite of the difference in volume measurements, the correlation between 3D echocardiography and MRI assessment of the right ventricle ejection fraction (RVEF) is quite strong [17]. All in all, echocardiography can be very useful, provided that a complex standard protocol is followed.

2. Anatomy and physiology of the right ventricle

The RV has an anterior position in the chest and lies immediately behind the sternum. It has a triangular or crescent shape and three distinct regions with different embryological origin and electrophysiological properties. The three regions include: 1) the inlet component, 2) the apical trabecular component and 3) the outlet component [18]. The inlet component extends from the tricuspid valve insertion to the level of the papillary muscle, surrounding and supporting the tricuspid valve and the subvalvular apparatus. The trabecular component extends from the papillary muscles level to the apex and contains coarse trabeculations. The inlet and trabecular components have a common embryological origin and form a morphological and functional structure called sinus. The sinus is the pivot structure for RV contraction. The outlet component, also called the infundibulum, conus or the RV outflow tract (RVOT) has its distinct embryological origin and is functionally different from the sinus. This component has a smooth surface and a minute contribution to RV output volume, and is the last cardiac structure to be activated, at end systole [19]. This region is particularly important in patients with congenital heart disease [20] and arrhythmias such as the idiopathic outflow tachycardia [21], as well as for the diagnosis of arrhythmogenic right ventricle dysplasia (ARVD), for which the left parasternal long-axis view is usually preferred [22]. All in all, each region of the RV (Figure 1) is essential in patients with cardiopulmonary disorders and should be analysed in correlation with segmental coronary vascularisation [18, 23].

RV physiology is closely linked to its anatomical properties. The thin, trabeculated free wall is adapted to the low pressures in the pulmonary circulation, its dynamics being very different from that of the LV. RV contraction is generated by the progression of a peristaltic wave which begins at the inlet and moves towards the infundibulum. RV depolarization triggers the

http://dx.doi.org/10.5772/55832

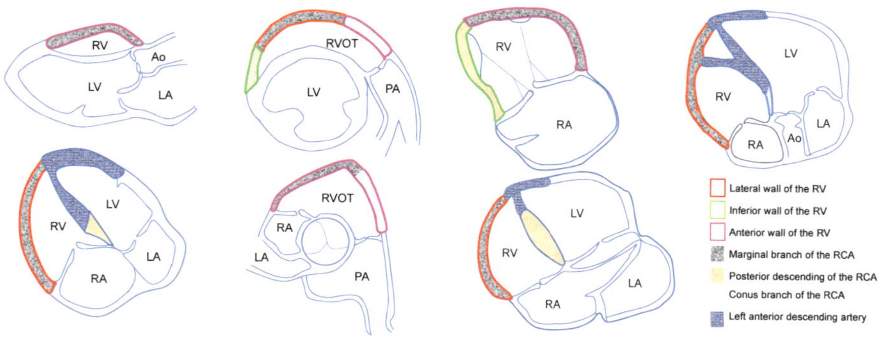

Figure 1. Segmental anatomy of right ventricle in correlation with segmental coronary vascularisation. Adapted from Rudski et al. [23]. RV=right ventricle; RVOT= right ventricular outflow tract; RA=right atrium; RCA=right coronary artery; PA=pulmonary artery; LV=left ventricle; LA=left atrium.

mechanic activity which consists of inward, longitudinal and circumferential traction; the systolic function is mainly determined by the longitudinal contraction which causes the shortening of the ventricle, with equal contribution from the interventricular septum and the free wall [24]. Several factors contribute to RV global function, namely the preload, afterload and contractility. The preload is dependant on the volume status, the tricuspid valve gradient and the venous return from the vena cava. The afterload is determined by the resistance opposed by the pulmonary valve, the pulsatile flow reflected from the main pulmonary artery, the impedance of the proximal pulmonary artery and arterioles [25]. Pulmonary vascular resistance may not, therefore, be used to assess RV total afterload, particularly in patients with pulmonary hypertension [25]. Due to its thin free wall and high compliance, the RV can easily adapt to increased preload by dilatation, which can be well tolerated for a long time, although it eventually leads to RV failure. By contrast, elevated afterload is poorly tolerated from an early stage, as the RV has little capacity for compensatory hypertrophy, which is quickly followed by increased stiffness and chamber dilatation [3]. In clinical practice, changes in preload and afterload alter RV contraction. Other factors that may impair RV systolic function include abnormal variations of the heart rate, pharmacological agents, or ventricular interdependence [25]. Ventricular interdependence refers to the fact that the shape, size and compliance of one ventricle may influence the shape, size or pressures in the other ventricle, an essential concept for understanding the pathophysiology of RV dysfunction [9].

3. Assessment of right chambers morphology and systolic function

3.1. Echocardiography

Echocardiography can help with qualitative morphological examination by 2D and 3D echocardiography. Although 2D echocardiography is widely applied in everyday clinical practice for the morphological and functional assessment of cardiac chambers and valves, 3D echocardiography is more accurate in assessing chamber volumes, mass and functions and provides a superior view of the valves. 2D echocardiography of the right chambers may provide diameter, area and volume measurements, which should be indexed to body surface, and allows the assessment of the systolic pulmonary artery pressure (sPAP) using the tricuspid regurgitation flow and inferior vena cava (IVC) diameter and its variations during the respiratory cycle. Newer techniques, such as tissue Doppler and strain-rate imaging, provide valuable data on the systolic and diastolic functions of the RV.

3.1.1. Right ventricle

A complete evaluation of RV structure should include the study of RV volume, shape and internal architecture, RV hypertrophy and mass, tissue characterization, assessment for potential masses [8], and regional wall motion abnormalities [26]. Normally, the RV has a crescent shape when viewed from the parasternal short-axis incidence; when the RV is submitted to pressure and volume overload, the crescent shape changes to a D shape, with subsequent septal flattening, leading to impaired LV filling and decreased output. Septal movement analysis can help distinguish between RV volume and pressure overload; in the case of volume overload, septal flattening only occurs during the diastole, whereas, in the presence of pressure overload, it is persistent throughout the entire cardiac cycle [27-28]. This phenomenon is quantitatively analyzed by deriving the eccentricity index, calculated as the RV anteroposterior over the RV septolateral diameter ratio (which may be measured at end-systole or end-diastole); a value>1 suggests RV overload and was shown to be positively correlated with pulmonary artery hypertension [29].

a. Acquisition and measurements:

Although qualitative assessment of the RV has its virtues, quantitative assessment provides more accurate and interpretable data. Morphology assessment may include diameter, area and volume measurements. RV morphology should be assessed by 2D using several acoustic windows such as the parasternal long-axis view (which allows RV anterior wall visualisation), the parasternal short-axis view (to assess the infundibulum and some of the RV anterior wall), the left parasternal RV inflow window (for the anterior, lateral and inferior RV walls, depending on the section level), the subcostal view (for the lateral wall and the infundibulum), the apical 4-chamber view, and apical 5-chamber view (for assessment of the RV lateral wall) [26] (Figure 2). Usually, the RV is best measured at end-diastole using the 4-chamber apical view. From this window, three dimensions can be derived: the basal diameter (the largest diameter in the basal third of the RV, usually just below the tricuspid annulus); the medial diameter (measured at the level of the LV papillary muscles); the longitudinal diameter (measured from the RV apex to the tricuspid annulus plane). RV free wall thickness is best measured from the subcostal view at the end of the diastole, using either 2D or M-mode imaging techniques; oblivious of the preferred method, measurements should exclude trabeculations, the papillary muscle, and the pericardium. RV volume and function may also be assessed by 3D transthoracic echocardiography using apical and subcostal views. Usually, four-beat images are necessary to include the entire RV, although newer techniques allow a good evaluation using a single beat, at the expense of temporal and spatial resolution [26].

http://dx.doi.org/10.5772/55832

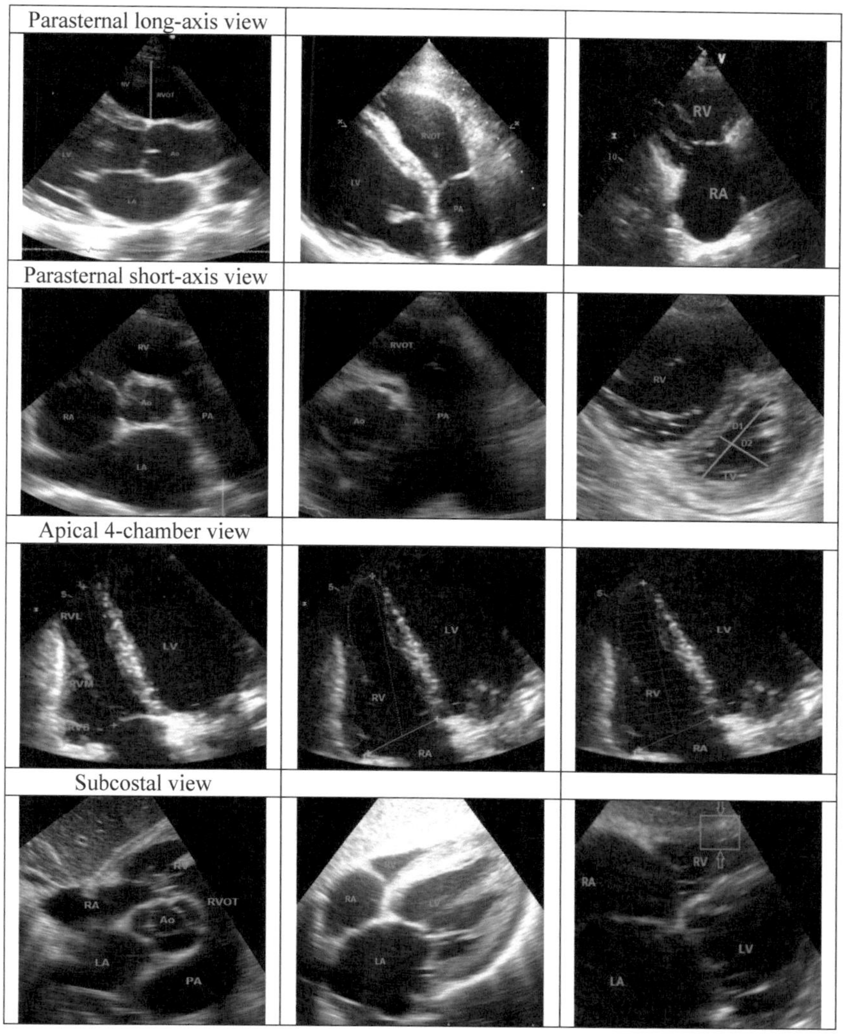

Figure 2. Echocardiography 2D views for right ventricle chamber.

Images are available for off-line analysis, allowing accurate endocardial contours delineation and RV volumes measurement from sequential long axis planes. End-diastolic measurements are taken at the peak of the R wave of QRS complexes, while end-systolic volumes are measured in the first frame before opening of the tricuspid valve [26]. Furthermore, trabeculations are included in the blood pool. The end-diastolic, end-systolic RV and stroke volume, as well as RVEF and RV mass are calculated using Simpson's rule.

b. Qualitative values:

An empirical comparison of LV and RV dimensions allows RV description as (Table 1): normal (when the RV has smaller dimensions when compared to the LV, with RV apex more basal than the LV apex); mildly dilated (when the RV is enlarged, but still smaller than the LV);

moderately dilated (when the RV and LV dimensions are equal); severely dilated (when the RV is larger than the LV) [30]. However, normal values have been established for quantitative assessment: a basal diameter >42 mm, a median diameter >35 mm and a longitudinal diameter >86 mm indicate RV dilatation. The parasternal short-axis view of the great vessels allows RVOT measurement at the level of the pulmonary valve insertion (the distal diameter) for which a value of >27 mm signifies RV dilatation. Proximal RVOT diameter can be measured from either the long or the short-axis parasternal views, with a normal maximum value of 33 mm. However, the former is usually preferred, as it is more reproducible [23]. RV areas are measured at end-diastole and end-systole, with the following normal values: RV end-diastole area 20.1 ± 4 cm^2 and RV end-systole area 10.9 ± 2.9 cm^2 [26, 30]. RV volumes may be calculated by using either the Simpson method or the area-length method and normal values range between 63-103 mL for end-diastolic volumes and 22-56 mL for end-systolic volume [31]. However, these 2D echocardiography measurements were proved to be inaccurate by comparison with 3D echocardiography and cardiac MRI derived volumes. Normal thickness ranges from 3 to 5 mm [23], and any value surpassing 5 mm suggests RV hypertrophy, which is usually a response to pressure overload, in the absence of associated pathology, such as infiltrative or hypertrophic cardiomyopathies [23].

2D echocardiography	**Reference values**	**Mildly dilated**	**Moderately dilated**	**Severely dilated**
RV dimensions				
Basal RV diameter (RVD1), mm	20-28	29-33	34-38	"/>39
Mid-RV diameter (RVD2), mm	27-33	34-37	38-41	"/>42
Base-to-apex length (RVL), mm	71-79	80-85	86-91	"/>92
RVOT diameters				
Above aortic valve, (RVOT proximal) mm	25-29	30-32	33-35	"/>36
Above pulmonic valve (RVOT distal), mm	17-23	24-27	28-31	"/>32
RV area				
RV diastolic area, cm^2	11-28	29-32	33-37	"/>38
RV systolic area, cm^2	7.5-16	17-19	20-22	"/>23
RV volume				
RV diastolic volume, mL	63–103			
RV systolic volume, mL	22–56			

Table 1. Reference limits and partition values of right ventricular size

The lack of accuracy in assessing RV volumes by 2D echocardiography is mainly determined by the complex RV geometry and the heavily trabeculated inner wall contour. Real 3D echocardiography overcomes these limitations and provides a superior evaluation of ventricular volume, mass and function, as well as a more complete view of the valves [26]. Moreover, 3D echocardiography was proved to be a reliable noninvasive modality of directing the bioptome to the desired site of biopsy within the RV. In one study, 3D echocardiography provided accurate anatomic details and was proved to allow sufficient pulmonary valve visualization in 68% of the patients and an excellent RVOT visualisation in 40% [32]. Normal medium values of RV end-diastolic and end-systolic volumes were established at 49 ± 10 and 16 ± 6 mL/m^2 respectively, with a mean RVEF of 67 ± 8% [33]. Another study provided normal reference ranges of indexed volumes: 38.6 to 92.2 mL/m^2 for RV end-diastolic volume, 7.8 to 50.6 mL/m^2 for end-systolic volume, 22.5 to 42.9 mL/m^2 for stroke volume in women and higher values in men: 47.0 to 100 mL/m^2 for RV end-diastolic volume, 14.2 to 48.4 mL/m^2 for end-systolic volume, and 23.0 to 52.6 mL/m^2 for stroke volume [34].

c. Clinical Application

The structural assessment of the RV provides information concerning the pressure and volume loading conditions which may lead to functional impairment. The RV gradually adapts to pressure overload by hypertrophy and interventricular septal flattening, with systolic function impairment, RV and tricuspid annulus enlargement and aggravated tricuspid regurgitation, which trigger RV diastolic dysfunction. Therefore, RV morphology should be assessed periodically in patients with acute or chronic respiratory pathology and valvulopathies with the purpose of identifying early anomalies which might be corrected by a proper therapeutic approach. Until recently, the eccentricity index was based on measurements made from the parasternal short-axis view, at the level of papillary muscles. However, one recent study shows that these measurements were less accurate than those made at the apical level, which was superior in terms of correlation with aggravated pulmonary hypertension [35], right chamber dilatation and RV systolic dysfunction [36]. In addition to that, ultrasound imaging techniques may identify regional morphologic abnormalities that occur in ARVD, provided the area of dysplasia is large enough. The diagnosis of ARVD is likely in the presence of significant local wall aneurysm (major diagnostic criterion), trabeculation disarray, increased thickness of the moderator band, with hyperechogenic appearance and RVOT dilatation [37]. However, despite the advantages, the diagnosis of ARVD by imaging techniques cannot rely on echocardiography alone.

3.1.2. Right atrium

The RA has its own complex pathology, as it responds to both RV volume and pressure overload. In addition to that, RA enlargement was documented in patients with atrial arrhythmias such as atrial fibrillation by both 2D and 3D echocardiography; moreover, it has been proven that RA remodelling occurs in atrial fibrillation and regresses if sinus rhythm is restored and maintained after radiofrequency catheter ablation [38]. However, RA dilatation is most often encountered in patients with elevated pulmonary hypertension.

a. Acquisition and measurements:

The RA is most often visualized from the apical 4-chamber view or the subcostal view [23, 26, 39]. However, due to the fact that standardized data concerning RA assessment is scarce, current evaluation includes exclusively RA minimum and maximum diameter and RA area estimation. All these measurements are made by planimetry from the apical 4-chamber view, at the end of the ventricular systole, when the atrium volume is largest (Figure 3). 3D echocardiography, although time consuming, may also be employed to calculate RA volume, with the advantage of more accurate endocardial border tracing at end-systole. To this purpose, two orthogonal planes (two-plane), four equiangular planes (four-plane), and eight equiangular planes (eight-plane) may be used [40]. All the collected data can be analyzed on and off-line, with cropping and threshold processing. The final result depends on the accurate and complementary use of these processing tools [41].

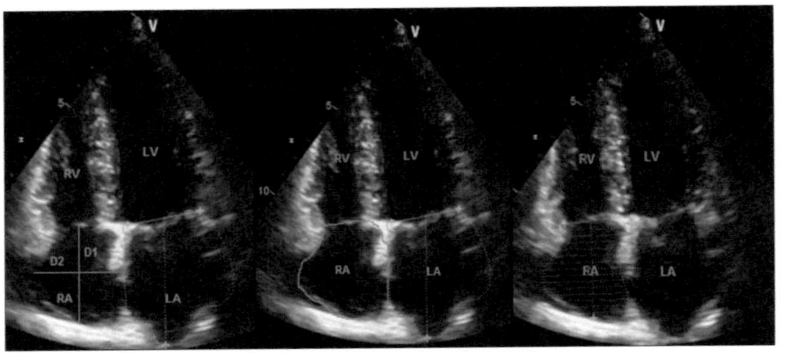

Figure 3. Echocardiography 2D views for right atrium.

b. Qualitative values:

The maximal short-axis distance is measured at mid level, with an upper reference limit of 44 mm. The maximal long axis distance is measured from the center of the tricuspid annular plane to the center of the RA superior wall, describing a straight line parallel to the interatrial septum; the threshold for the maximal normal value has been established at 53 mm [23] (Table 2). RA area provides a more accurate assessment, but it is more time-consuming and, thusly, avoided by most physicians. The upper reference limit has been established at 18 cm^2 or at 9 cm^2/m^2. The normal RA volume indexed to body surface area is 34 mL/m^2 for men and 27 mL/m^2 for women [26, 36].

2D echocardiography	Reference values	Mildly dilated	Moderately dilated	Severely dilated
RA dimensions				
RA minor-axis dimension, mm	29-45	46-49	50-54	"/>55
RA minor-axis dimension/BSA, mm/m^2	17-25	26-28	29-31	"/>22

Table 2. Reference limits and partition values for right atrium 2D dimensions

In 3D echocardiography, RA volumes are calculated using the following formula: 0.85 (D^2)/L, where D is the area in the four-chamber view and L the vertical long-axis [42]. Images should be taken from three different beats and the loops and tracings from the first examination should be available during the second and third examination to improve accuracy (Table 3) [42].

RA 3D echocardiography	Men	Women
RAEF, %	46-74	48-83
RAVI max, mL/m^2	18-50	17-41
RAVI min, mL/m^2	7-22	5-18

Table 3. Reference limits and partition values for right atrium 3D dimensions

c. Clinical Application

Real-time 3D echocardiography is believed to be a more reproducible and robust method for atrial volume measurements than 2D echocardiography [42], particularly in the presence of pathological conditions such as pulmonary disorders, congenital heart disease, valvular disease, and heart failure.

3.1.3. Inferior vena cava

Right chamber and pulmonary artery pressure assessment also relies on inferior vena cava (IVC) diameter measurement and the study of its variation during the respiratory cycle. In normal subjects, the IVC collapses, reducing its diameter with more than 50% after a sniff [43]; during a spontaneous, normal breathing cycle, changes in pleural pressure occur, which influence RA pressure; while inbreathing, the intrathoracic pressure becomes lower, allowing a more significant venous return and a decrease in IVC diameter. Respiratory variations are abolished in case of cardiac tamponade or severe right heart failure [43].

a. Acquisition and measurements:

The subcostal 4-chamber view is used to measure the IVC at end-expiration, proximal to the emergence of the hepatic veins, which is usually located at 0.5 to 3 cm of the IVC-RA ostium. Maximum and minimum diameters should be measured perpendicular to the long axis of the IVC. Measurements may be facilitated by using M-mode (Figure 4).

b. Qualitative values:

Current guidelines [23] established an upper reference limit of 21 mm for IVC diameter. For an IVC diameter ≤21 mm and an inbreathe variation of >50%, the RA pressure is estimated at 3 mmHg (range 0 – 5 mmHg). If IVC diameter is >21 mm, and the inbreathe collapse is lower than 50%, the RA pressure is estimated at 15 mmHg (range, 10 – 20 mmHg). However, some cases do not fit this paradigm; in that situation, if IVC >21 mm and significant collapse (>50%) occurs after a sniff, or if IVC ≤21 mm, but there is scarcely any inbreathe diameter variation or none at all, RA pressure is estimated at 8 mmHg (Table 4). Other authors [44] have previously suggested a different approach (Table 4). The reference normal value interval for the IVC diameter was set at 15 – 25 mm; if the measured IVC diameter remained within these limits, and decreased with >50% after a sniff, the RA pressure was estimated at 5 – 10 mmHg; if inbreathe variation was <50%, RA pressure was estimated at 10 – 15 mmHg, and at 15 – 20 mmHg if IVC diameter was greater than 25 mm. If IVC was dilated and remained flat during the respiratory cycle, and dilated hepatic veins were also visualized, RA pressure was considered to be >20 mmHg.

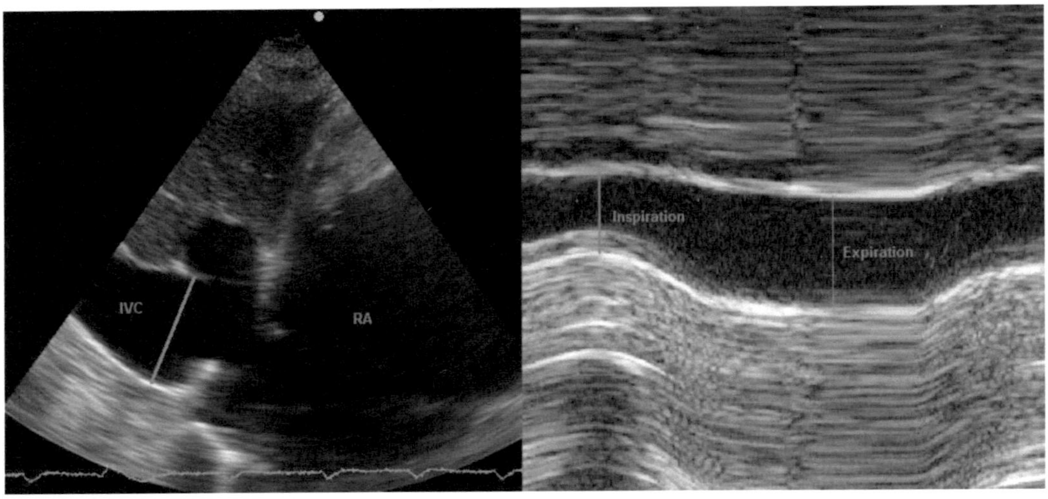

Figure 4. Measurement and view of the inferior vena cava (IVC) perpendicular to the long axis at end-expiration, just proximal to the junction of the hepatic veins that lie proximal to the ostium of the right atrium.

IVC diameter	Change after "sniff"	Estimated right atrium pressure (mmHg)
	Estimated right atrium pressure by Rudski [23]	
≤ 21 mm	Collapse "/>50%	3 mmHg (range 0 – 5 mmHg)
"/> 21 mm	Collapse <50%	15 mmHg (range 10 – 20 mmHg)
"/>21 mm	Collapse "/>50%	8 mmHg (range 5 – 10 mmHg)
≤ 21 mm	Collapse <50%	8 mmHg (range 5 – 10 mmHg)
	Estimated right atrium pressure by Otto [43]	
Normal range (15–25 mm)	Collapse "/>50%	5 – 10 mmHg
Normal range (15–25 mm)	Collapse <50%	10 – 15 mmHg
Dilated ("/>25 mm)	Collapse <50%	15 – 20 mmHg
Dilated ("/>25 mm)	Flat	"/> 20 mmHg

Table 4. Right atrium pressure assessment by inferior vena cava collapse and inbreathe variation

http://dx.doi.org/10.5772/55832

c. Clinical Application

Oblivious of the approach, estimated RA pressure is added to the tricuspid regurgitation gradient in order to calculate the systolic pulmonary artery pressure (sPAP). Usually, IVC diameter is only used to assess sPAP, and is not interpreted individually. However, one study focused on idiopathic pulmonary hypertension patients showed that an IVC diameter ≥20 mm, with respiratory variation <50%, was a prognostic factor for mortality [45]. In some cases, such as young athletes, dehydrated patients or in the presence of mechanical respiratory assistance devices, IVC diameter correlates poorly with RA pressure.

3.1.4. Right ventricle systolic function

Assessing RV systolic function can be difficult, due to the particular morphology of the RV. Geometrical assumptions are based on pyramidal and ellipsoidal models which are not particularly accurate, as the RV has a rather irregular shape. Moreover, area and volume estimation can be impaired by the presence of trabeculations in the RV, which should be excluded from myocardial border tracings. For volume calculation, area-length and disk summation (Simpson's) methods are used, the latter being more accurate. However, volumes are underestimated by 2D echocardiography [46], when compared to 3D echocardiography [47] and cardiac MRI [34]. Cardiac computed tomography may also be used, but RV volumes tend to be overestimated using this imaging technique [48], while cardiac MRI remains the gold standard for RV assessment, although it was shown to correlate very well with real-time 3D echocardiography measurements [11]. These imaging techniques are often unavailable in most centres, rendering 2D echocardiography quite important, despite its downfalls. A complete 2D echocardiography examination should include area and volume assessment, as well as several derived parameters (Table 5), such as right ventricle fractional area change (RVFAC) and the RVEF, tricuspid annular plane systolic excursion (TAPSE), systolic velocity of the myocardium (St wave) and right ventricular myocardial performance index (RVMPI).

2D echocardiography	Reference values	Mildly dilated	Moderately dilated	Severely dilated
RVFAC, %	32-60	25-31	18-24	<17
RVEF, %	43–65	40-30	30-20	<20
TAPSE, mm	15-20	13-15	10-12	<10

Table 5. Reference limits and partition values of right ventricular systolic function as measured in the apical 4-chamber view

a. Right ventricle fractional area change

The RVFAC is estimated using the formula: (end-diastolic area – end-systolic area)/end-diastolic area x 100, with a lower reference value for normal RV systolic function of 35% [23] and was previously proved to diminish in primary pulmonary hypertension patients, when compared to healthy controls [49] (Figure 5). Normal RVFAC and partition values [30] are shown in Table 5. In one study, RVFAC was found to be an independent predictor of heart failure, stroke and higher mortality in patients with prior myocardial infarction [50].

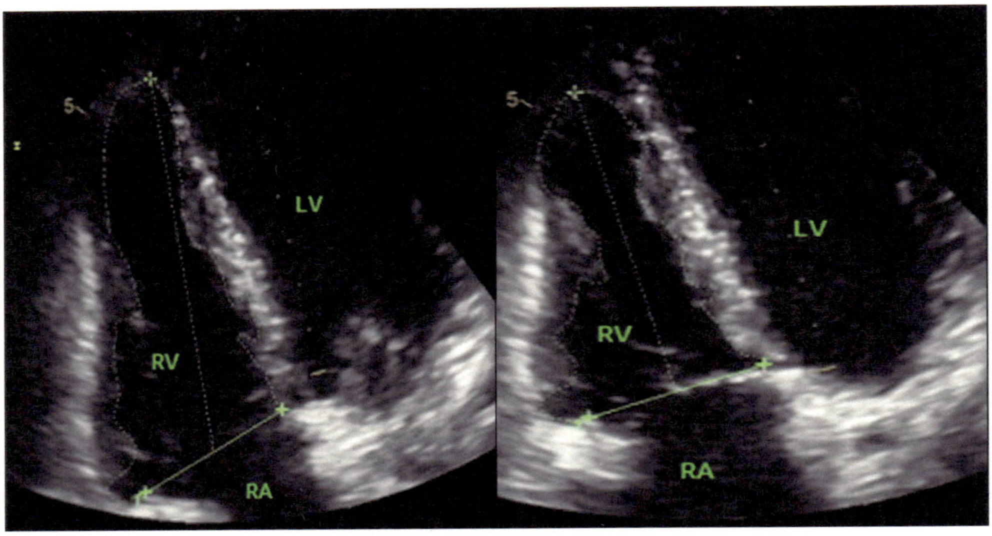

Figure 5. Measurement of the right ventricular fractional area change (RVFAC), views for right ventricle chamber.

b. Right ventricular ejection fraction

The RVEF is derived using the formula: (end-diastolic volume – end-systolic volume)/end-diastolic volume, for which the minimal normal value was established at 44% (Figure 6). Although RVEF measurement by echocardiography is impaired by geometrical assumptions, difficult endocardial border tracing and the fact that the RVOT is not included in area and volume assessment, it is still a valuable parameter, as some studies showed that RVEF is a strong and independent predictor of mortality in heart failure [51-52]. Both RVFAC and RVEF were proved to significantly correlate with other RV function parameters such as the myocardial performance index [53]. As mentioned above, the RV systolic function is dependent on the LV function and can be altered in the presence of interventricular septum movement abnormalities. The LV systolic function is mostly determined by the radial contraction, while the thin RV free wall systolic movement is predominantly determined by longitudinal shortening.

c. Tricuspid annular plane systolic excursion

To assess RV free wall systolic shortening, the TAPSE is measured. This parameter is assessed using the apex-4-chamber view and the M-mode; the cursor is placed at the level of the tricuspid annular plane, allowing the examiner to assess the base to apex motion of the annular plane during systole (Figure 7). The minimal reference threshold has been established at 16 mm (normal values ranging around 22 ± 4 mm) and it is inferred that higher TAPSE values correspond to a better systolic function. TAPSE is easy to measure, reproducible, does not

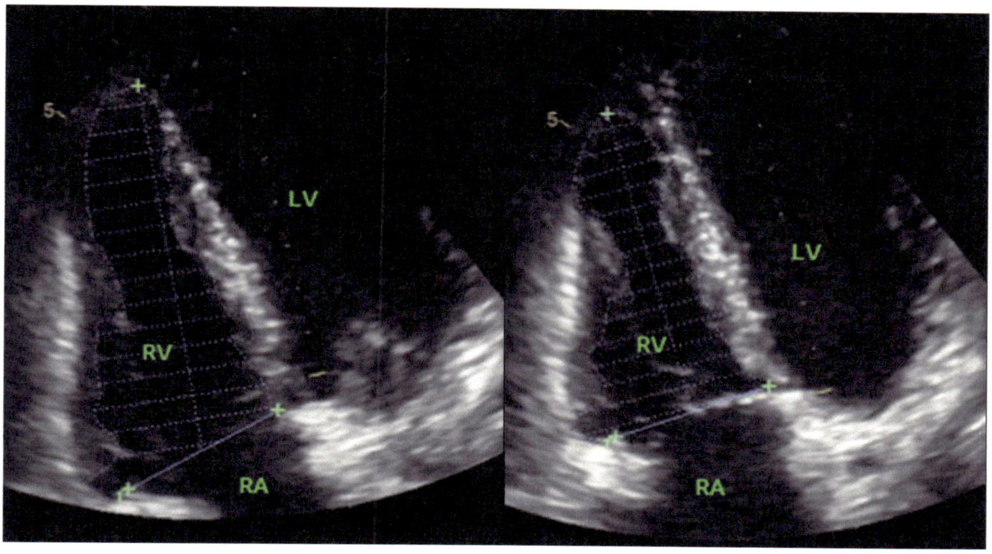

Figure 6. Measurement of the right ventricular ejection fraction (RVEF), views for right ventricle chamber.

require special equipment and is valuable when assessing RV function after myocardial infarction, but does present with some downfalls, particularly due to the fact that it only reflects the basal segment function, ignoring other regions. Moreover, it is angle and load dependant. However, some studies have shown that it correlates well with RVFAC and Simpson's method derived RVEF [35, 54], as well as ventriculography derived RVEF [24] and that it is highly reliable as a prognostic tool in pulmonary hypertension [52, 55], heart failure [24] and dilated cardiomyopathy, oblivious of the ischemic or non-ischemic aetiology [52].

Some level of correspondence has been demonstrated between TAPSE (in mm) and RVEF; a TAPSE of 5 mm corresponds to a 20% RVEF, 10 mm to a 30% RVEF, 15 mm to 40%, 20 mm to 50% [56].

d. Tissue Doppler analysis

Tissue Doppler imaging's (TDI) may be used to obtain other indices of RV performance such as the St wave, the isovolumic contraction velocity and the derived myocardial acceleration (Figure 8) during isovolumic contraction. All these parameters are quite independent of anatomical properties and do not rely on any geometrical assumptions, but may be influenced by load conditions. As they are angle dependent, Doppler beam alignment should be optimal. The isovolumic contraction velocity is measured using either pulsed or colour-coded TDI with sample volume placement on the RV free wall at the level of the tricuspid annulus. The isovolumic contraction phase starts immediately after the A′ wave corresponding to ventricular filling during atrial systole and precedes the St wave which describes ventricle wall movement during the ejection phase. In one study, the isovolumic contraction velocity was shown to correlate very well with mean RA pressure and proved to have 100% sensitivity and 78% specificity for a cut-off value <6 cm/s [57-58].

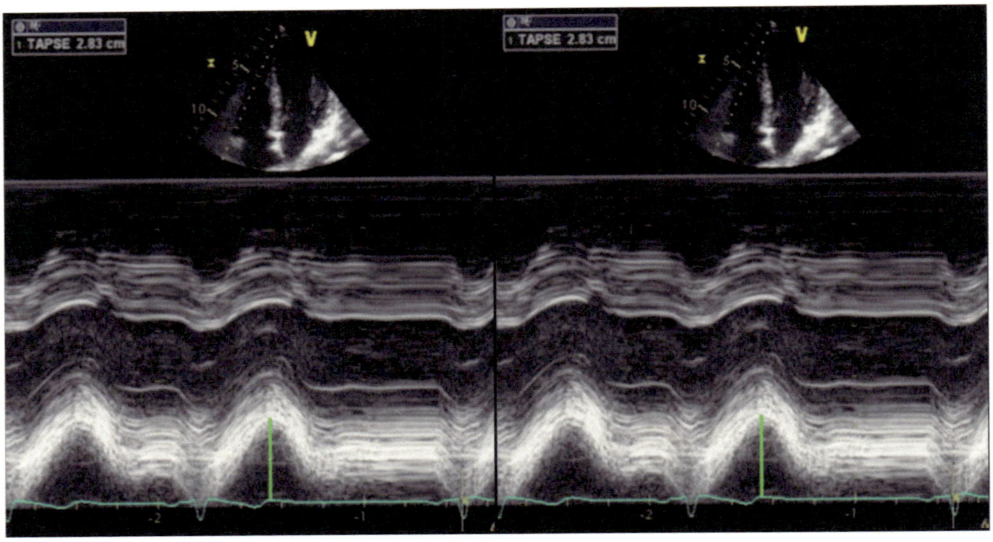

Figure 7. Measurement of the tricuspid annular plane systolic excursion (TAPSE) in normal and pulmonary artery hypertension individual, in the four chamber view a straight line (M mode) is drawn through the lateral tricuspid valve annulus.

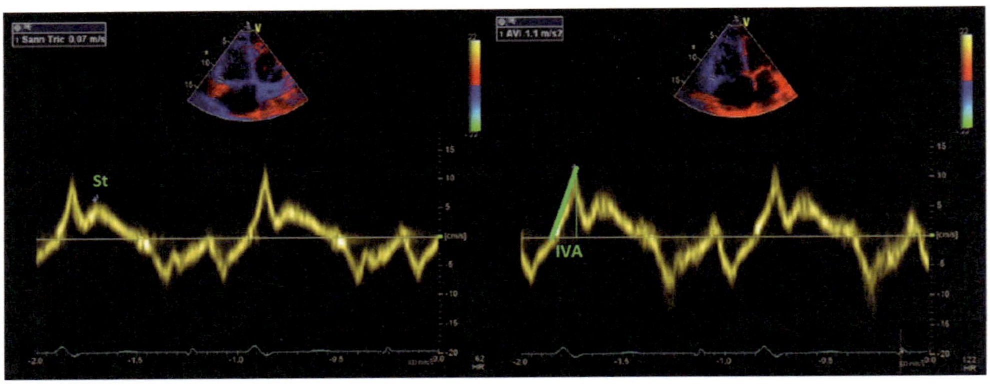

Figure 8. Pulsed wave tissue Doppler with the sample placed at the level of the tricuspid annulus of the RV free wall, demonstrating peak systolic velocity (St), and myocardial acceleration during isovolumic contraction (IVA).

This parameter may further be used to derive the myocardial acceleration during isovolumic contraction (IVA) which is calculated as the peak isovolumic contraction velocity divided by the time to peak velocity. Myocardial acceleration during isovolumic contraction may be measured either by pulsed-wave TDI or colour-coded TDI, but normal values seem to be different; in one study, values proved to be up to 20% higher when assessed by pulsed-wave TDI, by comparison with colour-coded TDI evaluation [23] [59]. In addition to that, normal values vary with age [60] and heart rate. For tissue Doppler assessment, pooled data from 10 studies established a lower reference value of 2.2 m/s [23]. IVA was studied on several animal models which lead to significant conclusions which may be implemented in every day practice.

Vogel et al. conducted a study on pigs, proving that IVA is afterload and preload independent [61], while Hashimoto et al. conducted their research on sheep, proving that IVA correlates very well with peak positive dp/dt measured invasively by right heart catheterization [62]. In humans, studies have shown that IVA was significantly correlated with disease severity in patients with chronic obstructive pulmonary disease [63], obstructive sleep apnoea [64], RV remodelling triggered by type 2 diabetes mellitus [65], and that it may be used for early detection of RV dysfunction in patients with mitral stenosis [66] or systemic sclerosis, even before the onset of pulmonary hypertension [67]. Moreover, in one study on patients who underwent corrective surgery for transposition of the great arteries, IVA was proved to be superior to the peak systolic myocardial velocity in assessing the reduction of functional reserve, in both the RV and LV [68].

TDI may also be used for measuring the highest St wave. This parameter is obtained from the apical four chamber view by positioning the sample volume either at the level of the tricuspid annulus, on the lateral wall, or in the middle or apical segments segment. The latter locations are, however, avoided by most physicians as adequate signals are rarely obtained and measurements are less reproducible, with greater interobserver variability [58]. St may be measured using pulsed tissue or colour coded TDI, and is, as other TDI parameters, angle dependent, but less influenced by loading conditions or RV anatomy when compared to other systolic function parameters. Mean annular velocities have been established at 8.5 – 10 cm/s, while basal free wall velocities are slightly higher at 9.3 – 11 cm/s [23], with lower velocities in elderly subjects due to the increased stiffness of the myocardium [60, 69, 70]. The main limitation of this parameter is determined by the fact that it only reflects changes in systolic movement of the basal segment which are extrapolated as descriptive for the systolic function of the entire RV. This type of measurement may sometimes be inaccurate in the presence of segmental RV systolic dysfunction which may occur in some clinical conditions such as RV myocardial infarction, ARVD or pulmonary embolism. A St value under 10 cm/s should rise suspicion of RV dysfunction, especially in young subjects, although a minimum reference value was established at 6 cm/s by pooled data from several studies [23]. In one research, a St value of <12 cm/s showed high sensitivity (81%), specificity (82%) and negative predictive value (92%) for the diagnosis of RV myocardial infarction [71], while Meluzin et al. demonstrated it was significantly correlated with RVEF and that a value <11.5 cm/s predicted RV systolic dysfunction with 90% sensitivity and 85% specificity in patients with heart failure [72]. Also, St was also shown to be lower, as expected, in patients with systemic sclerosis [67].

e. Right ventricular myocardial performance index

Both the systolic and diastolic functions of the RV may be evaluated using the myocardial performance index, also known as RVMPI or Tei index. This index can be obtained either by pulsed Doppler or TDI and is defined by the ratio of isovolumic time/ejection time. The ejection time is assessed by placing the pulsed Doppler cursor at the level of the RVOT and is measured from the onset to the cessation of the systolic pulmonary artery flow. When the pulsed Doppler cursor is placed at the level of the tricuspid annulus, the time from the cessation of the A wave to the onset of the next E wave is measured and the difference between this interval and the ejection time signifies the total isovolumic time (isovolumic resting time + isovolumic contraction time). These measurements are taken from two different acoustic windows and, implicitly, in different points in time, therefore errors can occur if the RR interval is not regular. Consequently, measurements may only be made if the rhythm is regular and are not feasible in case of atrial fibrillation. When using the TDI method, measurements are taken during a single heart beat, by placing the cursor at the level of the tricuspid annulus (Figure 9). The isovolumic contraction time (IVCT) is measured from the cessation of the At wave to the beginning of the St wave, the ejection time (ET) – from the onset to the cessation of the St wave, and the isovolumic relaxation time (IVRT) – from the end of the S′ wave to the onset of the Et wave. The correlation between the tissue Doppler and pulsed Doppler methods are modest, due to differences in isovolumic times, which lead to higher cut-off points when tissue Doppler is used, as it was shown in studies focused on the LV [73, 74]. Moreover, one recent study showed that LV Tei index assessment by tissue Doppler was better correlated with the LV ejection fraction in patients with heart failure [75]. Similar results were obtained in a study on a paediatric population with congenital heart disease which showed that the TDI derived Tei index values were different from those obtained by pulsed Doppler and that they had additional utility, as they might help differentiate systolic from diastolic dysfunction by providing specific information on the isovolumetric intervals [76]. For the RVMPI, the upper reference limit has been established at 0.40 by the pulsed Doppler method and at 0.55 by the tissue Doppler method [23]. Any values above these thresholds are considered to be pathological, as stated by Brierre et al. who obtained a mean value of the Tei index of 0.90 in their research on idiopathic pulmonary artery hypertension patients; moreover, they showed that values ≥0.98 were associated with increased mortality [45].

Up to date, RVMPI was proved to be useful for RV function assessment in several studies. One study on patients with acute RV myocardial infarction showed that the Tei index was valuable for diagnosis, RV function quantification and, interestingly, for acute improvement assessment [77].

In another research by Blanchard et al. conducted on patients with chronic thromboembolic pulmonary hypertension, RVMPI was shown to be a valuable tool for monitoring disease severity and for assessing outcome after pulmonary thrombo-endarterectomy, and positively correlated with pulmonary vascular resistance, measured by right heart catheterization [78]. Moreover, RVMPI was shown to be a high sensitivity and specificity parameter for diagnostic purposes in patients with acute pulmonary embolism, as well as a valuable tool for assessing the response to efficient anticoagulant therapy [79-81]. In addition to that, Haddad et al. demonstrated that both the RVMPI and the RVFAC may have an incremental prognostic value in terms of mortality and morbidity after valvular heart surgery [82], while others confirmed its utility in assessing global RV function in children with congenital heart disease [83-84]. The Tei index also proved its value in RV function assessment in patients with sleep apnoea, as it was positively correlated with the anoxia-hypoxia index, while RVFAC showed inverse correlation with the same parameter [85].

The echocardiographic evaluation of RV by RVMPI has many advantages, as it is non-invasive, widely available, reproducible and independent of any geometric assumptions. If the pulsed wave Doppler method is used, errors may occur if the RR interval is variable. This downfall may, however, be limited by using the tissue Doppler method which allows measurement taking during a single heart beat, but results are still unreliable in patients with atrial fibrillation. Other disadvantages include load dependency and altered results when RA pressure is elevated, due to artificial IVRT shortening which leads to lower RVMPI values [86].

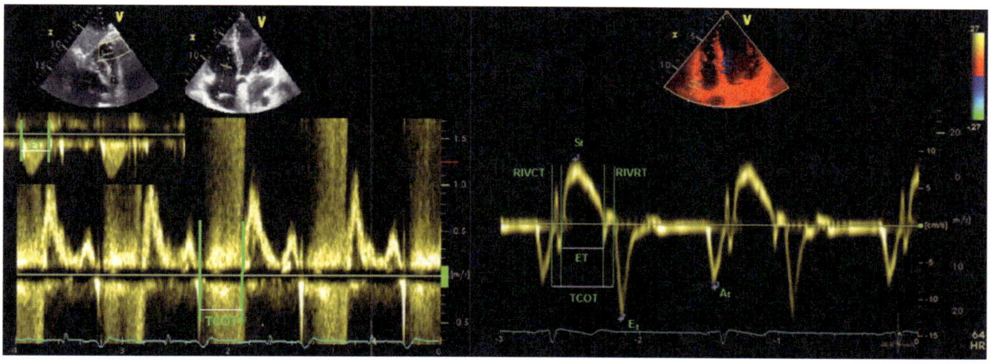

Figure 9. Measurement of right ventricular myocardial performance index (RVMPI) by pulsed wave Doppler of tricuspid regurgitation and tissue Doppler with the sample placed at the level of the tricuspid annulus of the RV free wall.

f. Analyzing the tricuspid regurgitation flow

RV systolic function assessment can also be performed by analyzing the tricuspid regurgitation flow, which is commonly visualized from the apical 4-chamber view. Using continuous-wave Doppler, several parameters can be derived, such as: RV-RA pressure gradient, systolic, diastolic and mean pulmonary artery pressure (sPAP; dPAP; mPAP), the rate of pressure rise in the RV (dp/dt), and the previously described right index of myocardial performance (RVMPI). To this purpose, an optimal parallel alignment of the continuous Doppler cursor to the tricuspid regurgitation (TR) flow should be obtained. The rate of pressure rise in the RV (dp/dt) was first described in 1962 and measured invasively by right heart catheterization. An echocardiographic method based on the Bernoulli equation was developed to serve the same purpose, although it was shown that continuous-wave Doppler analysis of the TR flow significantly underestimated peak RV pressures when compared to invasive measurements [87]. The rate of pressure rise is calculated by measuring the time interval in which the tricuspid flow velocity rises from 1 m/s to 2 m/s (Figure 10). Based on the Bernoulli equation, this rise in velocity corresponds to a pressure elevation of 12 mmHg. Other researchers suggest that dp/dt assessment correlates better with invasive measurements if the studied time interval is focused on a rise in velocity from 0.5 to 2 m/s, which corresponds to a 15 mmHg rise in pressure [88]. The value of dp/dt is expressed in mmHg/sec, but normal reference values have not been established so far; this parameter, although easy to obtain, has limited clinical value, also due to the fact that it is load and angle dependent. However, values <400 mmHg/s are likely to be abnormal [23]. One small study showed that the dp/dt over maximum RV pressure ratio had a significant correlation to the NYHA functional class, while dp/dt by itself had none at all [89]. Nowadays, this parameter is of little interest.

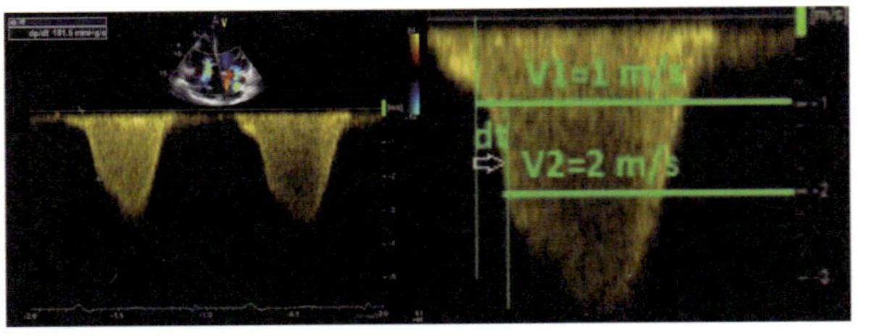

Figure 10. Measurement of the rate of pressure rise in the ventricles (dp/dt) of tricuspid regurgitation in the four chamber view in pulmonary artery hypertension individual.

The RV-RA pressure gradient may also be estimated using the peak velocity of the TR flow based on the simplified Bernoulli equation: peak pressure gradient of TR= 4 x (TR maximum velocity)^2. As it is angle dependant, the best possible alignment of the continuous-wave Doppler cursor with the regurgitation jet should be obtained and several measurements, from several acoustic windows (most often, apical 4 chamber view and parasternal RV inflow view), should be taken (Figure 11). The signal with the highest velocity and density should be used; the Doppler signal may be enhanced by injecting agitated saline into the venous flow. Moreover, special attention is necessary to exclude RVOT obstruction, which often occurs in congenital heart disease. sPAP is then calculated by adding the estimated RA pressure (assessed by IVC diameter and its inbreathe variations, as described above) to the RV-RA gradient.

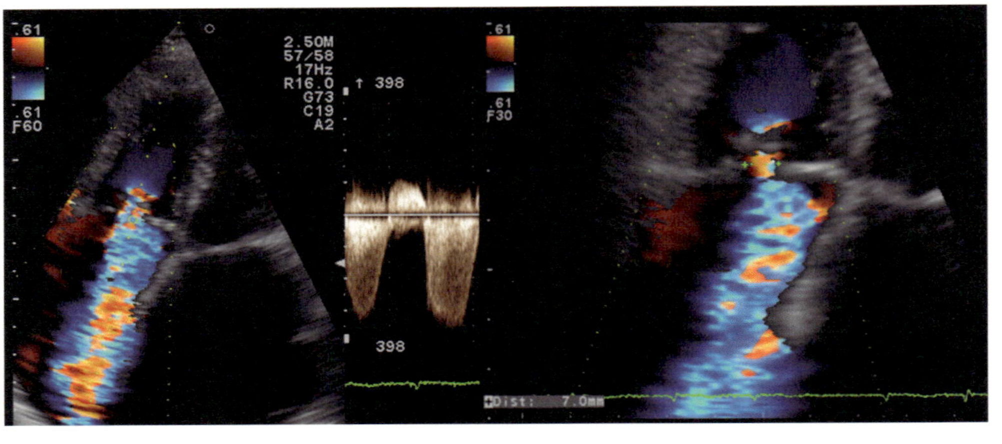

Figure 11. Doppler echocardiographic determination of systolic pulmonary artery pressure (sPAP).

A tricuspid regurgitation jet maximum velocity of ≤ 2.8 m/s renders pulmonary hypertension unlikely, a velocity of >3.4 m/s – likely, while values between 2.8 m/s and 3.4 m/s indicate that pulmonary hypertension is possible [90-91]. Normal resting values have been established at ≤36 mmHg for peak systolic pressure, assuming a RA pressure of 3-5 mmHg [23, 92].

The severity of pulmonary hypertension may be underestimated in the presence of severe tricuspid regurgitation that leads to elevated RA pressure and, consequently, to a lesser RV-RA pressure gradient and lower sPAP (Table 6).

	TR maximum velocity	PAPs	Other echo parameters suggesting HTP*
PH unlikely	≤ 2.8 m/s	≤ 36 mmHg	
PH possible	≤ 2.8 m/s	≤ 36 mmHg	+
	2.9 – 3.4 m/s	37 – 50 mmHg	+/-
PH likely	>3.4 m/s	>50 mmHg	

* dilated right chambers; increased thickness of the RV free wall; abnormal shape and function of the interventricular septum; dilated pulmonary artery; increased velocity of the pulmonary regurgitation jet; short acceleration time of RV ejection in the pulmonary artery; PH - pulmonary hypertension

Table 6. Arbitrary criteria for the presence of pulmonary hypertension based on continuous Doppler derived systolic pulmonary artery pressure (sPAP) and tricuspid regurgitation (TR) jet maximum velocity [90].

Like the sPAP, the dPAP can be derived by applying the Bernoulli equation to the pulmonary regurgitation flow: dPAP=4 x (end-diastolic regurgitant velocity)^2 + RA pressure. The pulmonary regurgitation flow may also be used to calculate the mPAP pressure after the same principle, by the formula mPAP= (4 x early PR velocity) + RA pressure, or by adding RA pressure to the velocity time integral (VTI) of the tricuspid regurgitation, the latter method being the most accurate, as it correlates better to invasive measurements by right heart catheterization [93, 94]. Previous methods relied on more vague estimations, based on the sPAP and dPAP: mPAP= 1/3 sPAP + 2/3 dPAP, or obtained by analysing the pulmonary artery continuous wave Doppler flow, using the formula mPAP= 79 – (0.45 x AT) (AT= acceleration time) [95].

The AT is measured from the onset of the pulmonary flow, which corresponds to the onset of the QRS complex on the ECG, to the onset of the maximum pulmonary velocity; consequently, the shorter the AT, the higher the mPAP. This formula applies when the heart rate is between 60 and 100 bpm, and the AT is below 120 msec. A study showed, however, that, in case of aggravated pulmonary hypertension, when AT shortens below this threshold, the formula mPAP= 90 – (0.62 x AT) led to more accurate results [95]. Despite the technical progress and reasonable mathematical and physical assumptions, right chamber and pulmonary pressure assessment by echocardiography is not sufficient for diagnosing pulmonary hypertension. In pulmonary artery hypertensive patients, right heart catheterisation remains the golden standard [94], as it is needed to confirm the diagnosis, to assess severity and to test for vessel reactivity if specific therapy is considered [90]. Several studies have shown that sPAP is considerably underestimated by echocardiography when compared to right heart catheterization, oblivious of the used method [96-98]. However, despite all the limitations, the assessment of pulmonary artery pressures by echocardiography can be used as a screening method for pulmonary hypertension [90, 94].

g. Regional RV Strain and Strain Rate

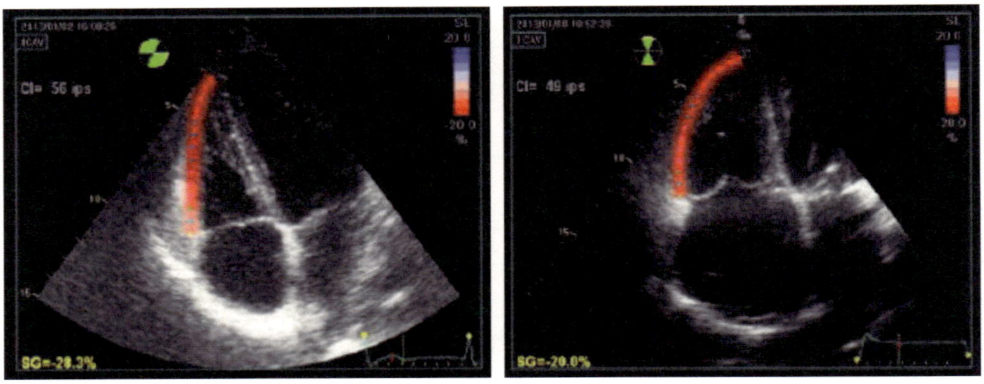

Figure 12. Measurement of global right ventricular deformation by speckle-tracking with the sample placed at the level of the RV free wall in normal and pulmonary artery hypertension individual.

Strain and strain rate (SR) imaging can provide valuable data on the relative deformation of myocardial segments under stress. The resting length of the myocardium (L0) changes when submitted to a certain force (L1). Myocardial strain is best described by the L1-L0/L0 ratio, expressed in a certain percentage, which is negative when shortening occurs and positive when the myocardium lengthens. The SR can be derived using strain and the velocity of myocardial deformation, expressed in 1/s. The particular anatomy of the RV, which is mainly composed of longitudinal and oblique fibres, renders it highly susceptible to strain variations at lower stress when compared to the LV [99]. Right myocardial velocities are, thusly, higher than in the LV and more elevated at the apex, when compared to the base, even in normal individuals [99].

TDI-derived and speckle-tracking echocardiography-derived strain and SR can be used to assess RV dynamics and were found to be both feasible and roughly comparable. Strain and SR correlate well with radionuclide RVEF [24].

Normal strain is 19 ± 6 % in the basal RV free wall, 27 ± 6 %, in the median and 32 ± 6 % at the apex for the prediction of RVEF >50% [100]. This renders strain assessment of the RV quite strenuous, with important limitations due to the need of perfect alignment of the TDI cursor to the rather thin free wall of the RV. In addition to that, strain analysis is highly dependent on hemodynamic variations [101]. In patients with RV disease or dysfunction, peak systolic strain and SR are significantly reduced and delayed compared with individuals with normal RV function [24].

RV speckle-tracking is less challenging in terms of angle issues, provided that optimal endocardial border tracking is performed [102]. In 2D speckle-tracking analysis, a certain selected zone is studied in motion, allowing a good assessment of the longitudinal, radial and torsion movements of the RV (Figure 12); however, this method is limited by a low temporal resolution [102].

h. 3D echocardiography

3D echocardiography may also be used to assess right ventricle systolic and diastolic functions. It has been previously demonstrated that 3D echocardiography-derived RVEF correlated negatively with 2D-derived pulmonary arterial systolic pressure and positively with TAPSE, the peak systolic velocity, and the fractional shortening area [32]. In one study, patients with mitral valve prolapse who underwent surgical treatment had significantly lower TAPSE and peak systolic velocities of the tricuspid annulus after surgery, while 3D-derived RVEF remained the same (58.4 ± 4%) [32]. Moreover, 3D echocardiography analysis was used to describe RV systolic function in patients with various cardiovascular disorders, showing that patients with pulmonary hypertension had the largest RV volumes and RVEF, while those with idiopathic dilated cardiomyopathy had considerably lower RVEF when compared to patients with valvular heart disease [32].

In another study, normal RVEF reference values were established at 38.0% to 65.3% for women and 29.9% to 58.4% for men [34].

3.2. Cardiac magnetic resonance imaging

Nowadays, cardiac MRI is considered to be the gold standard for determining RV volume and function [11]. This method should be taken into account when 3D echocardiography is not sufficient for evaluation.

a. Acquisition and measurements:

Cardiac MRI requires a minimum 1.5 Tesla scanner, with a phased-array cardiac coil. Cine imaging acquired 2-chamber and 4-chamber views allow the positing of a retrospectively ECG-gated steady-state free procession pulse sequence using following parameters: repetition time 3.5–4.2 ms, echo time 1.5–1.8 ms, flip-angle 45°, matrix 256 × 256, field of view 250–350 mm, slice thickness 5–8 mm with a gap of 0–2 mm depending on body size; 12 slices should be acquired [10]. Cardiac MRI allows an accurate delineation of the endocardial and epicardial borders in all planes and all cardiac phases; in addition to that, the systolic descent and twist of the tricuspid valve is quantified by tracking of the valve motion on the long-axis cines in order to correct for loss of systolic RV volume due to AV ring descent; thirdly, papillary muscles are delineated, with blood pool thresholding. This technique allows the calculus of RV end-systolic and end-diastolic volumes, RV ejection fraction and right ventricular mass with a great degree of precision [103-104]. Cardiac MRI allows a complete assessment of the RV inflow and outflow, regardless of ventricular size or shape. The extent of myocardial damage or fibrosis is evaluated using late gadolinium enhancement.

b. Qualitative values:

Several reference values for RV volumes have been mentioned, with significant gender differences; consequently, larger RV volumes were documented in males when compared to females: RV end-diastolic volume 190 ± 33 mL vs. 148 ± 35 mL, RV end-systolic volume 78 ± 20 mL vs. 56 ± 18 mL [105]. Other values were obtained in another study, which compared MRI-derived volumes against 3D echocardiography volumes, proving the former were larger. The following mean normal values were established for RV end-diastolic, end-systolic, and stroke volumes: 134.2 ± 39.2 mL vs. 124.0 ± 34.4 mL; 69.7 ± 25.5 mL vs. 65.2 ± 23.5 mL; and 64.5 ± 24.1 mL vs. 58.8 ± 18.4 mL [106].

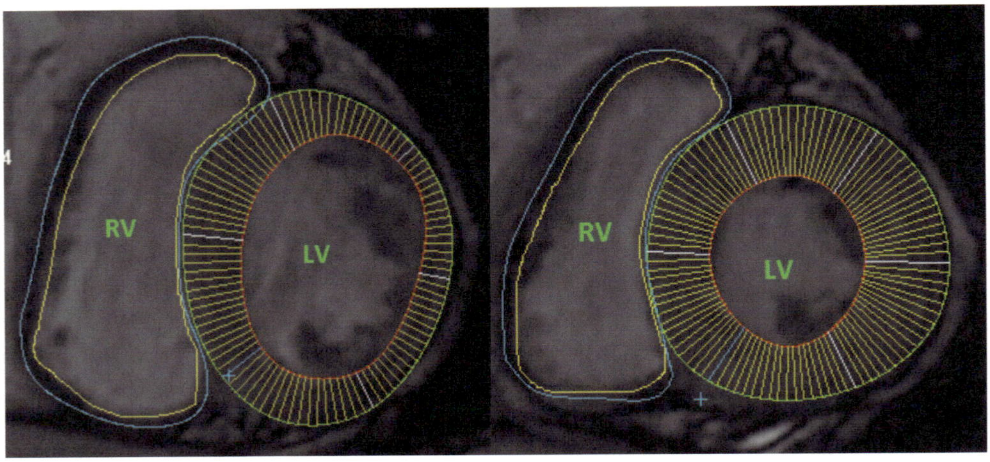

Figure 13. Cardiac MRI steady-state free procession sequence for the assessment of right ventricular function en-diastolic and en-systolic. RV=right ventricle; LV=left ventricle.

c. Clinical Application

The efficiency of 3D echocardiography vs. cardiac MRI in RV assessment was compared in many studies. One research group conducted a study on 60 pulmonary artery hypertensive patients [4], proving that 3D echocardiography had some advantages over cardiac MRI, as it could be routinely used for serial imaging and at the bedside. Moreover, it was previously shown that both 3D echocardiography and cardiac MRI may be used to assess RV remodeling in pulmonary artery hypertension patients [11, 34, 107]. However, cardiac MRI results proved to be more reproducible in terms of assessing RV ejection fraction and RV mass [26]. Although less available, cardiovascular MRI is frequently used nowadays to describe RV systolic function; recent imaging techniques allow a good assessment of parameters such as ventricular volumes, ejection fraction, and myocardial mass, with increased accuracy when compared to echocardiography. Stroke volumes, cardiac output, and volumes routed through cardiac shunts can be derived using flow velocities and cross sectional areas. These methods are similar to those used in Doppler echocardiography, but provide a better accuracy, as MRI velocity analysis can be conducted in any orientation or plane. Tissue parameters are best visualized by contrast enhancement techniques (contrast-enhanced MRI), which typically use gadolinium-based magnetic contrast agents [103]. Similar to strain echocardiography, tagged MRI is used to study the 3-dimensional motion and deformation in the heart. Tags are regions of the myocardium, whose longitudinal magnetization has been altered before imaging which render them dark in MRI. These dark areas are landmarks within the heart which allow the detection of motion. In one study on patients with idiopathic pulmonary arterial hypertension, tagged MRI was used to identify significant interventricular asynchrony caused by a prolonged RV systolic contraction time, probably due to impaired electrical conductivity in the right ventricle. It was then showed that ventricular asynchrony led to impaired LV diastolic filling and, consequently, to decreased LV end-diastolic volumes [108]. Although further research would be needed to validate reproducible parameters for RV evaluation, echocar-

http://dx.doi.org/10.5772/55832

diography and cardiac MRI based techniques are, for the time being, of immense value. As mentioned before, cardiovascular MRI is nowadays considered to be the gold standard for RV assessment; in one research, some 3D echocardiography-derived measurements, such as the RVEF, compared well against cardiac MRI results, with little difference (47.8 ± 8.5% vs 48.2 ± 10.8%) [106]. However, in another study, a tendency to overestimate RVEF by 3D echocardiography, with a bias of approximately 13% (95% CI -52% to +27%), has been reported; moreover, in the same research, RV diastolic and RV systolic volumes were shown to be systematically and significantly underestimated by 3D echocardiography [109]. Solid correlations were established between 2D echocardiography tissue Doppler St wave velocity and MRI-derived RVEF [110]. In addition to that, it was shown that a systolic long-axis peak velocity of <11 cm/s at the lateral tricuspid annulus was associated with moderately impaired MRI-derived RVEF, while severely reduced RVEF ≤30% was best detected by RVMPI at a value of >0.50 [111].

4. Assessment of right ventricular diastolic dysfunction

4.1. Echocardiography

4.1.1. Tissue Doppler analysis

a. Acquisition and measurements:

The assessment of RV diastolic dysfunction strongly resembles LV evaluation. Validated parameters include the tricuspid flow E and A velocities, as well as the E/A ratio, the E wave deceleration time and the IVRT, which are assessed in a similar manner to mitral flow evaluation; the previously mentioned parameters are measured using the apical 4-chamber view by placing sample volume at the tips of the tricuspid leaflets.

Several limitations undermine the accuracy of tricuspid flow parameters, particularly the preload and afterload dependency. Preload variations are significant during the respiratory cycle due to fluctuant intrathoracic pressure, which is diminished during inbreathing and rises during expiration. Low intrathoracic pressure favours venous return to the RA, leading to better atrial filling and increased pressure; as a consequence, early diastolic ventricular filling is improved, with an increase in E wave velocity, while A wave velocities remain almost the same; subsequently, the E/A ratio may change. Conversely, lower E wave velocities are obtained when preload decreases during expiration. This is why some authors suggest that at least 5 beats should be analysed in each patient in order to obtain an average value that should have clinical significance [112]. Other physiological factors that influence tricuspid flow patterns are age, gender and tachycardia [112]. Measurements may also be altered by the presence of severe tricuspid regurgitation or atrial fibrillation [23]. Moreover, the thin-walled RV is also highly sensitive to afterload variations, particularly in patients with myocardial infarction or chronic ischemia [113]. TDI is another valuable tool for assessing RV diastolic function. TDI is used to measure velocities at the level of the tricuspid annulus (Et, At, Et/At) and to derive the E/Et ratio which is gaining interest as a marker of diastolic dysfunction. In clinical practice, both pulsed and colour TDI may be used; the former technique is simpler and provides a high temporal resolution, but is hindered by low spatial resolution [114]; the latter has high spatial resolution, but lower temporal resolution and provides mean velocities [115], as opposed to pulsed TDI, by which maximum velocities are measured. Although considered superior to pulsed wave Doppler techniques, TDI measurements have their limitations. Firstly, like pulsed Doppler parameters, they are influenced by age and gender [116].

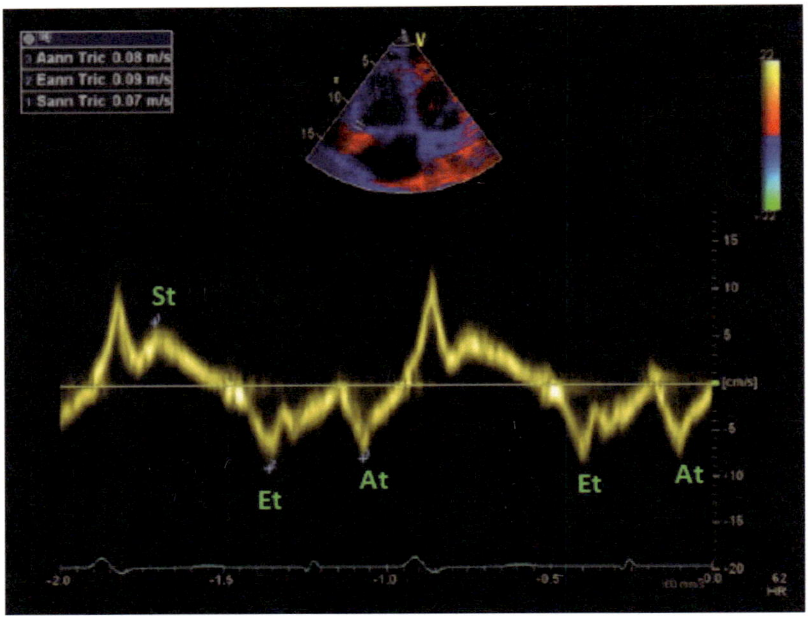

Figure 14. Pulsed wave tissue Doppler with the sample placed at the level of the tricuspid annulus of the RV free wall, demonstrating diastolic parameters (Et and At).

b. Qualitative values:

Moreover, although previous studies focused on the LV supported TDI load independency [117], Pelà et al. demonstrated in their research on healthy subjects that RV Et and At wave velocities were dependent on loading conditions; however, they also showed that Et and At velocity variations were proportional, and consequently, despite alterations in preload, the Et/At ratio remained constant. [118]. According to Horton et al., measuring parameters from ≥ 3 different beats during apnoea may reduce errors derived from load variations and the translational motion of the myocardium [119]. Despite the limitations, several researches have confirmed that pulsed and tissue Doppler allow a clinically significant evaluation of RV diastolic function. Puwanat et al. demonstrated that a tricuspid E/Et ratio >6 was associated with a mean right atrium pressure >10 mmHg in patients with heart failure and preserved ejection fraction [120]; this finding was consistent with data from a previous research by Utsunomyia et al. who demonstrated that intraatrial pressure assessment by use of the E/Et ratio was comparable with invasive hemodynamic measurements obtained by right heart catheterization and valuable as a prognostic tool for cardiovascular events in patients with chronic pulmonary artery hypertension [121] (Table 7).

Degree of diastolic dysfunction	Tricuspid E/A ratio	Additional parameters
Impaired relaxation	< 0.8	E/Et >6
Pseudonormal filling	0.8 – 2.1	diastolic flow predominance in the hepatic veins TDE < 120 msec
Restrictive filling	> 2.1	late systolic anterograde flow in the pulmonary artery

Table 7. Right ventricle diastolic dysfunction assessment

c. Clinical Application

As in the case of the left ventricle, RV diastolic function is the first to be impaired, preceding systolic dysfunction. Therefore, when RV impairment is suspected, diastolic function assessment is advised, as RV diastolic dysfunction has been confirmed as a marker of poor prognosis [23]. Most studies support the use of the following parameters: trans-tricuspid E/A ratio, E/E_t ratio, and RA size [23].

4.1.2. Color M-mode flow propagation velocity

a. Acquisition and measurements:

Color M-Mode flow propagation velocity (Vp) is most commonly measured by the slope method from the apical 4-chamber view, using color flow imaging with a narrow color sector; gain is adjusted to avoid noise. The M-mode cursor is placed at the center of the RV inflow blood column from the tricuspid valve to the apex. The color flow baseline is shifted to lower the Nyquist limit so that the central highest velocity jet is blue. Flow propagation velocity (Vp) is measured as the slope of the first aliasing velocity during early filling, measured from the tricuspid valve plane to 4 cm distally into the RV cavity. Alternatively, the slope of the transition from no color to color may be measured.

b. Qualitative values:

Vp values >50 cm/s are considered normal for the RV. The Et/Vp ratio varies proportionally with RA pressure, and may therefore be used either by itself, or in combination with IVRT to assess filling pressures. However, this rather challenging method is redundant in patients with decreased RV ejection fraction in which other parameters precisely identify diastolic dysfunction.

c. Clinical Application

The slowing of tricuspid-to-apical flow propagation measured by color M-mode Doppler is valuable in identifying diastolic dysfunction. In addition, it may help in assessing filling pressures when used in conjunction with tricuspid E. Essays were made to measure non-invasively the tricuspid-to-apical pressure gradient by color M-mode Doppler, but the method is not currently intended for routine clinical application, due to its difficulty. The non-invasive imaging assessment of the RV has gained raising interest and recent research has provided data which may improve standard clinical protocols. However, highly accurate reference values are yet to be established, and there are currently few available and reproducible parameters.

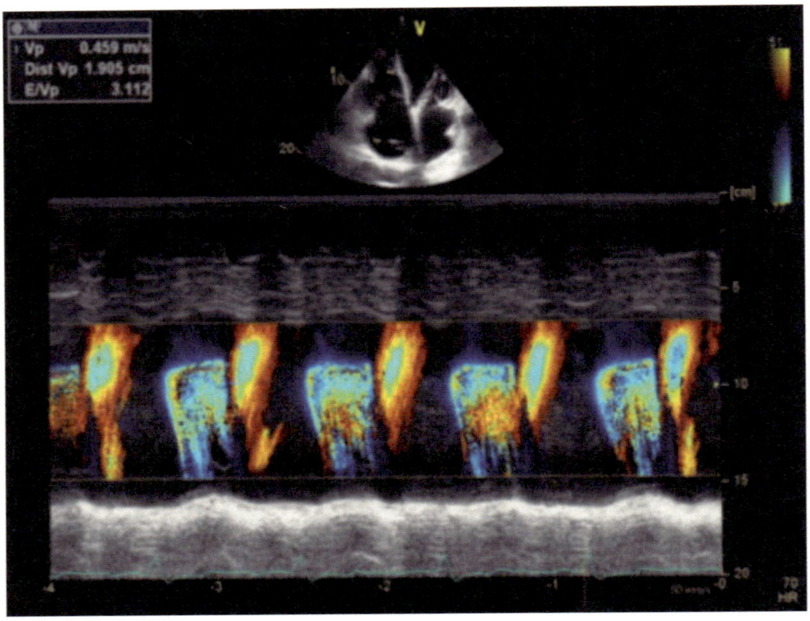

Figure 15. Pulsed color M-mode Vp imaging with the sample placed at the level of the tricuspid annulus of the RV free wall in pulmonary artery hypertension individual.

4.2. Cardiac magnetic resonance imaging

a. Acquisition and measurements:

The assessment of RV diastolic dysfunction by cardiac MRI is similar, as a principle, to the echocardiographic evaluation. 1.5 Tesla systems can be used to characterize the transtricuspid flow. To this purpose, 4-chamber views should be acquired. ECG-gated phase-contrast pulse sequences are positioned retrospectively, in a plane perpendicular to the transtricuspid inflow, at the level of the opened tricuspid tips, just bellow the tricuspid valve annulus. Two dynamic phase-contrast series, corresponding to an entire cardiac cycle, are acquired during breathhold: 1) the transtricuspid flow velocity sequence, and 2) a myocardial longitudinal velocity sequence. Due to technical progress, cardiac MRI is increasingly being used for blood and myocardial velocities assessment. In addition to that, several studies have demonstrated the usefulness of phase-contrast MRI for measuring diastolic function parameters [122]. However, these analyses are mostly based on manual positioning of regions of interest (ROIs) within the transtricuspid flow area or the myocardium on multiple phases [122, 123]. The derivative of the time/volume curve, expressed as peak filling rate is used to quantify diastolic function. The early and active peak tricuspid filling rates (PFR_E and PFR_A) and their ratio may be calculated [104].

b. Qualitative values:

Maceira et al [104] published the first normal ranges for MRI-derived RV diastolic function: PFR_E=371 mL/s, or 202 mL/m^2, PFR_A=429 mL/s, or 233 mL/m^2, PFR_E/PFR_E = 0.9 were significantly higher in males [104].

5. Hemodynamic assessment

As previously mentioned, Doppler echocardiography may be used for the non-invasive, indirect assessment of pulmonary artery pressures. To this purpose, the RV-RA pressure gradient is calculated by analyzing the tricuspid regurgitation flow and the obtained value is added to the estimated RA pressure; the latter is estimated by measuring the IVC and its collapsibility after a "sniff". The value of sPAP thusly derived is somewhat empirical. Several studies have shown that Doppler echocardiography systematically under- or overestimates pulmonary pressures, by comparison with direct, invasive measurements by right heart catheterization [96, 124].

Currently, right heart catheterization remains the gold standard for pulmonary artery pressure assessment, as it is necessary to confirm the diagnosis, assess hypertension severity and the reactivity to vasodilator agents [90]. Invasive measurements are particularly useful in patients with NYHA II and III heart failure who have mild pulmonary hypertension as assessed by echocardiography. In addition to that, right heart catheterization provides the advantage of vasoreactivity testing, which is compulsory before initiating vasodilator therapy and may help predict the response to treatment; nitric oxide, adenosine and epoprostenol are most commonly used for this purpose [90]. Patients who have an acute response to vasoreactivity testing are more likely to respond to long-tem therapy [125].

In conclusion, echocardiography may be used as a screening method, as it indicates the likelihood of pulmonary artery hypertension, rather than providing an actual diagnosis. Results should always be validated by right heart catheterization, particularly if specific vasodilator treatment is intended. All in all, 2D echocardiography has some limitations, some related to the empirical assessment of sPAP, others to the imprecision in chamber measurements due to geometrical assumptions or difficult endocardial border tracing. Presently, cardiac MRI is the golden standard in RV structure and function evaluation, due to its unlimited imaging planes, higher image resolution, and the ability to calculate volumes using three-dimensional measurements; however, cardiac MRI is seldom available in many centres, and hindered by prolonged acquisition and processing times. Moreover, its use is still limited in patients with implanted metallic devices, such as pace-makers, defibrillators, metallic prostheses or insulin pumps. Right heart catheterization allows a good evaluation of sPAP, but it is an invasive procedure and is not usually performed in the absence of other evidence of pulmonary artery hypertension. Standard 2D echocardiography is widely available, relatively cheap, does not present any risk for the patient, and may be performed even in the presence of metallic devices which would normally hinder an MRI examination. Although it only indicates the likelihood of pulmonary artery hypertension, it may be used to select candidates for right catheterization. In terms of assessing RV structure and function, further research would be needed in order to provide solid, reproducible parameters, with normal reference values.

Acknowledgements

This work was supported by grants 27020/24/2011 and 22714/2/2011 from the "Iuliu Hatieganu" University of Medicine and Pharmacy in Cluj-Napoca.

Author details

Lucia Agoston-Coldea[1] and Silvia Lupu[2]

*Address all correspondence to: luciacoldea@yahoo.com

1 The "Iuliu Hatieganu" University of Medicine and Pharmacy, Cluj-Napoca, Romania

2 The University of Medicine and Pharmacy of Targu Mures, Romania

References

[1] Kasimir, M.T, Seebacher, G, Jaksch, P, Winkler, G, Schmid, K, Marta, GM, Simon, P, & Klepetko, W. Reverse cardiac remodelling in patients with primary pulmonary hypertension after isolated lung transplantation. Eur J Cardiothorac Surg. (2004)., 26(4), 776-781.

[2] McLaughlin, V.V, Archer, S.L, Badesch, D.B, Archer, S.L, Badesch, D.B, Barst, R.J, Farber, H.W, Lindner, J.R, Mathier, M.A, McGoon, M.D, Park, M.H, Rosenson, R.S, Rubin, L.J, Tapson, V.F, & Varga, J. ACCF/AHA 2009 expert consensus document on pulmonary hypertension. J Am Coll Cardiol. (2009)., 53(17), 1573-1619.

[3] Badano, L.P, Ginghina, C, Easaw, J, Muraru, D, Grillo, M.T, Lancellotti, P, Pinamonti, B, Coghlan, G, Marra, M.P, Popescu, B.A, & De Vita, S. Right ventricle in pulmonary arterial hypertension: hemodynamics, structural changes, imaging and proposal of a study protocol aimed to assess remodelling and treatment effects. Eur J Echocardiogr. (2010)., 11(1), 27-37.

[4] Grapsa, J, O'Regan, D.P, Pavlopoulos, H, Durighel, G, Dawson, D, & Nihoyannopoulos, P. Right ventricular remodelling in pulmonary arterial hypertension with three-dimensional echocardiography: comparison with cardiac magnetic resonance imaging. Eur J Echocardiogr. (2010)., 11(1), 64-73.

[5] Kostrubiec, M, Kaczynska, A, & Pruszczyk, P. Right ventricle remodelling and elevated D-dimer concentration in patients 6 months after first episode of acute pulmonary embolism. Eur Heart J. (2008)., 29(16), 2059-2060.

[6] Mansi, T, Voigt, I, Leonardi, B, Pennec, X, Durrleman, S, Sermesant, M, Delingette, H, Taylor, A.M, Boudjemline, Y, Pongiglione, G, & Ayache, N. A statistical model for quantification and prediction of cardiac remodelling: application to tetralogy of Fallot. IEEE Trans Med Imaging. (2011)., 30(9), 1605-1616.

[7] Haddad, F, Doyle, R, Murphy, D.J, & Hunt, S.A. Right Ventricular Function in Cardiovascular Disease, Part II: Pathophysiology, Clinical Importance, and Management of Right Ventricular Failure. Circulation. (2008)., 117(13), 1717-1731.

[8] Haddad, F, Hunt, S.A, Rosenthal, D.N, & Murphy, D.J. Right Ventricular Function in Cardiovascular Disease, Part I: Anatomy, physiology, aging, and functional assessment of right ventricle. Circulation. (2008)., 117(11), 1436-1448.

[9] Haddad, F, Couture, P, Tousignant, C, & Denault, A.Y. The right ventricle in cardiac surgery, a perioperative perspective: I. Anatomy, Physiology, and Assessment. Anesth Analg. (2009)., 108(2), 407-421.

[10] Valsangiacomo Buechel, E.R, & Mertens, L.L. Imaging the right heart: the use of integrated multimodality imaging. Eur Heart J. (2012)., 33(8), 949-960.

[11] Niemann, P.S, Pinho, L, Balbach, T, Galuschky, C, Blankenhagen, M, Silberbach, M, Broberg, C, Jerosch-Herold, M, & Sahn, D.J. Anatomically oriented right ventricular volume measurements with dynamic three-dimensional echocardiography validated by 3-Tesla magnetic resonance imaging. J Am Coll Cardiol. (2007)., 50(17), 1668-1676.

[12] Martin, E.T, Coman, J.A, Shellock, F.G, Pulling, C.C, Fair, R, & Jenkins, K. Magnetic resonance imaging and cardiac pacemaker safety at 1.5-Tesla. J Am Coll Cardiol. (2004)., 43(7), 1315-1324.

[13] Juntilla, M.J, Fishman, J.E, Loperal, G.A, Pattany, P.M, Velasquez, D.L, Williams, A.R, Trachtenberg, B.H, Sanina, C, Mather, J, & Hare, J.M. Safety of serial MRI in patients with implantable cardioverter defibrillators. Heart. (2011)., 97(22), 1852-1856.

[14] Naehle, C.P, Strach, K, Thomas, D, Meyer, C, Linhart, M, Bitaraf, S, Litt ,H, Schwab, J.O, Schild, H, & Sommer, T. Magnetic Resonance Imaging at 1.5-T In Patients With Implanted Cardioverter Defibrillators. J Am Coll Cardiol. (2009)., 54(6), 549-555.

[15] Rosenthal, D, Chrisant, M.R, Edens, E, Mahony, L, Canter, C, Colan, S, Dubin, A, Lamour, J, Ross, R, Shaddy, R, Addonizio, L, Beerman, L, Berger, S, Bernstein, D, Blume, E, Boucek, M, Checchia, P, Dipchand, A, Drummond-Webb, J, Fricker, J,

Friedman, R, Hallowell, S, Jaquiss, R, Mital, S, Pahl, E, Pearce, F.B, Rhodes, L, Rotondo, K, Rusconi, P, Scheel, J, Pal Singh, T, & Towbin, J. International Society for Heart and Lung Transplantation: Practice guidelines for management of heart failure in children. J Heart Lung Transplant. (2004)., 23(12), 1313-1333.

[16] Crean, A, Ballard, G, Maredia, N, Greenwood, J.P, & Thomson, J.D. 3D echo systematically underestimates right ventricular volume compared to cardiac magnetic resonance in adult congenital heart disease patients with moderate or severe RV dilatation. J Cardiovasc Magn Reson. (2011)., 13, 78.

[17] van der Zwaan, H.B, Helbing, W.A, McGhie, J.S, Geleijnse, M.L, Luijnenburg, S,E, Roos-Hesselink, J.W, & Meijboom, F.J. Clinical value of real-time three-dimensional echocardiography for right ventricular quantification in congenital heart disease: validation with cardiac magnetic resonance imaging. J Am Soc Echocardiogr. (2010)., 23(2), 134-140.

[18] Ho, S.Y, & Nihoyannopoulos, P. Anatomy, echocardiography, and normal right ventricular dimensions. Heart. (2006)., 92 (suppl 1), i2-13.

[19] Chen, P.S, Moser, K.M, Dembitsky, W.P, Auger, W.R, Daily, P.O, Calisi, C.M, Jamieson S.W, & Feld, G.K. Epicardial activation and repolarization patterns in patients with right ventricular hypertrophy. Circulation. (1991)., 83(1), 104-118.

[20] Bashore TM. Adult congenital heart disease: right ventricular outflow tract lesions. Circulation. (2007)., 115(14), 1933-1947.

[21] Arya, A, Piorkowski, C, Sommer, P, Gerds-Li, J.H, Kottkamp, H, & Hindricks, G. Idiopathic outflow tract tachycardia: current perspectives. Herz. (2007)., 32(3), 218-225.

[22] Yoerger, D.M, Marcus, F, Sherill, D, Calkins, H, Towbin, J.A, Zareba, W, Picard, M.H. Echocardiographic findings in patients meeting task force criteria for arrhythmogenic right ventricular dysplasia: new insights from the multidisciplinary task study of right ventricular dysplasia. J Am Coll Cardiol. (2005)., 45(6), 860-865.

[23] Rudski, L.G, Lai, W.W, Afilalo, J, Hua, L, Handschumacher, M.D, Chandrasekaran, K, Solomon, S.D, Louie, E.K, & Schiller, N.B. Guidelines for the Echocardiographic Assessment of the Right Heart in adults: A Report fron the American Society of Echocardiography, a registered branch of the European Society of Cardiology, and the Canadian Society of Echocardiography. J Am Soc Echocardiogr. (2010)., 23(7), 685-713.

[24] Mor-Avi, V, Lang, R.M, Badano, L.P, Belohlavek, M, Cardim, N.M, Derumeaux, G, Galderisi, M, Marwick, T, Nagueh, SF, Sengupta, P.P, Sicari, R, Smiseth, O.A, Takeuchi M, Thomas, J.D, Vannan, M, Voigt, J.U, & Zamorano, J.L. Current and Evolving Echocardiographic Techniques for the Quantitative Examination of Cardiac Mechanics: ASE/EAE Consensus Statement on Methodology and Indications Endorsed by the Japanese Society of Echocardiography. Eur J Echocardiogr. (2011)., 12(3), 167-205.

[25] Brittain, E.L, Hemnes, A.R, Keebler, M, Lawson, M, Byrd, B.F, & DiSalvo, T. Right ventricular plasticity and functional imaging. Pulm Circ. (2012)., 2(3), 309-326.

[26] Grapsa, J, Dawson, D, & Nihoyannopoulos, P. Assessment of Right Ventricular Structure and Function in Pulmonary Hypertension. J Cardiovasc Ultrasound. (2011)., 19(3), 115-125.

[27] Feigenbaum, H, Armstrong, W, & Ryan, T. Left atrium, right atrium, right ventricle. In: Feigenbaum H (ed.) Feigenbaum's echocardiography. 6th ed. Philadelphia: Lippincot, Williams and Wilkins. (2005)., 181-213.

[28] Ryan, T, Petrovic, O, Dillon, J.C, Feigenbaum, H, Conley, M.J, & Armstrong, WF. An Echocardiographic Index for Separation of Right Ventricular Volume and Pressure Onverload. J Am Coll Cardiol. (1985)., 5(4), 918-924.

[29] López-Candales, A, Rajagopalan, N, Kochar, M, Gulyasy, B, & Edelman, K. Systolic eccentricity index identifies right ventricular dysfunction in pulmonary hypertension. Int J Cardiol. (2008)., 129(3), 424-426.

[30] Lang, R.M, Bierig, M, Devereux, R.B, Flachskampf, F.A, Foster, E, Pellikka, P.A, Picard, M.H, Roman, M.J, Seward, J, Shanewise, J.S, Solomon, S.D, Spencer, K.T, Sutton, M.S, & Stewart, W.J. Recommendations for chamber quantification: a report from the American Society of Echocardiography's Guidelines and Standards Committee and the Chamber Quantification Writing Group, developed in conjunction with the European Association of Echocardiography, a branch of the European Society of Cardiology. J Am Soc Echocardiogr. (2005)., 18(12), 1440-1463.

[31] Kovalova, S, Necas, J, & Vespalec, J. What is a "normal" right ventricle? Eur J Echocardiogr. (2006)., 7(4), 293-297.

[32] Gillam, L.D, & Otto, C.M. Advanced Approaches in Echocardiography. Philadelphia: Elsevier Inc. Saunders. (2012).

[33] Tamborini, G, Marsan, N.A, Gripari, P, Maffessanti Brusoni, D, Muratori, M, Caiani, E.G, Fiorentini, C, & Pepi, M. Reference values for right ventricular volumes and ejection fraction with real-time three-dimensional echocardiography: evaluation in a large series of normal subjects. J Am Soc Echocardiogr. (2010)., 23(2), 116-126.

[34] Gopal, A.S, Chukwu, E.O, Iwuchukwu, C.J, Katz, A.S, Toole, R.S, Schapiro, W, & Reichek, N. Normal Values of Right Ventricular Size and Function by Real-time 3-Dimensional Echocardiography: Comparison with Cardiac Magnetic Resonance Imaging. J Am Soc Echocardiogr. (2007)., 20(5), 445-455.

[35] Lopez-Candales, A, Dohi, K, Rajagopalan, N, Edelman, K, Gulysasy, B, & Bazaz, R. Defining normal variables of right ventricular size and function in pulmonary hypertension: an echocardiographic study. Postgrad Med J. (2008)., 84(987), 40-45.

[36] Lopez-Candales, A, Bazaz, R, Edelman, K, & Gulyasy, B. Apical Systolic Eccentricity Index: A Better Marker of Right Ventricular Compromise in Pulmonary Hypertension. Echocardiogr. (2010)., 27(5), 534-538.

[37] Frances RJ. Arrhythmogenic right ventricle dysplasia/cardiomyopathy. A review and update. Int J Cardiol. (2006)., 110(3), 279-287.

[38] Muller, H, Noble, S, Keller, P.F, Sigaud, P, Gentil, P, Lerch, R, Shah, D, & Burri, H. Biatrial anatomical reverse remodeling after radiofrequency catheter ablation for atrial fibrillation: evidence from real-time three-dimensional echocardiography. Europace. (2008)., 10(9), 1073-1078.

[39] Wang, Y, Gutman, J.M, Heilbron, D, Wahr, D, & Schiller, NB. Atrial volume in a normal adult population by two-dimensional echocardiography. Chest. (1984)., 86(4), 595-601.

[40] Quraini, D, Pandian, N.G, & Patel, A.R. Three-dimensional echocardiographic analysis of right atrial volume in normal and abnormal hearts: comparison of biplane and multiplane methods. Echocardiogr. (2012)., 29(5), 608-613.

[41] Faletra, F.F, Ho, S.Y, & Auricchio, A. Anatomy of Right Atrial Structures by Real-Time 3D Transesophageal Echocardiography. JACC Cardiovasc Imaging. (2010)., 3(9), 966-975.

[42] Aune, E, Baekkevar, M, Roislien, J, Rodevand, O, & Otterstad, J.E. Normal reference ranges for left and right atrial volume indexes and ejection fractions obtained with real-time three-dimensional echocardiography. Eur J Echocardiogr. (2009)., 10(6), 738-744.

[43] Jardin, F, & Vieillard-Baron, A. Ultrasonographic examination of the venae cavae. Intense Care Med. (2006)., 32(2), 203-206.

[44] Otto CM. Textbook of clinical Echocardiography. 3rd Edition. Philadelphia: Elsevier Saunders. (2004)., 154-159.

[45] Brierre, G, Blot-Souletie, N, Degano, B, Tetu, L, Bongard, V, & Carrie, D. New echocardiographic prognostic factors for mortality in pulmonary arterial hypertension. Eur J Echocardiogr. (2010)., 11(6), 516-522.

[46] Hudsmith, L.E, Petersen, S.E, Francis, J.M, Robson, M.D, & Neubauer, S. Normal human left and right ventricular and left atrial dimensions using steady state free precession magnetic resonance imaging.J Cardiovasc Magn Reson. (2005)., 7(5), 775-782.

[47] Shiota T. 3D echocardiography: evaluation of the right ventricle. Curr Opin Cardiol. (2009)., 24(5), 410-414.

[48] Sugeng, L, Mor-Avi, V, Weinert, L, Niel, J, Ebner, C, Steringer-Mascherbauer, R, Bartolles, R, Baumann, R, Schummers, G, Lang, R.M, & Nesser, H.J. Multimodality Com-

parison of Quantitative Volumetric Analysis of the Right Ventricle. JACC Cardiovasc Imaging. (2010)., 3(1), 10-18.

[49] Raymond, R.J, Hinderliter, A.L, Willis, P.W, Ralph, D, Caldwell, E.J, Williams, W, Ettinger, N.A, Hill, N.S, Summer, W.R, De Boisblanc, B, Schwartz, T, Koch, G, Clayton, L.M, Jobsis, M.M, Crow, J.W, & Long, W. Echocardiographic predictors of adverse outcomes in primary pulmonary hypertension. J Am Coll Cardiol. (2002)., 39(7), 1214-1219.

[50] Anavekar, N.S, Skali, H, Bourgoun, M, Ghali, J.K, Kober, L, Maggioni, A.P, McMurray, J.J, Velazquez, E, Califf, R, Pfeffer, M.A, & Solomon, S.D. Usefulness of right ventricular fractional area change to predict death, heart failure, and stroke following myocardial infarction (from the VALIANT ECHO study). Am J Cardiol. (2008)., 101(5), 607-612.

[51] Meluzin, J, Spinarova, L, Hude, P, Krejci, J, Kincl, V, Panovsky, R, & Dusek, L. Prognostic importance of various echocardiographic right ventricle functional parameters in patients with symptomatic heart failure. J Am Soc Echocardiogr. (2005)., 18(5), 435-444.

[52] Ghio, S, Gavazzi, A, Campana, C, Inserra, C, Klersy, C, Sebastiani, R, Arbustini, E, Recusani, F, & Tavazzi L. Independent and additive prognostic value of right ventricular systolic function and pulmonary artery pressure in patients with chronic heart failure. J Am Coll Cardiol. (2001)., 37(1), 183-188.

[53] Zimbarra Cabrita, I, Ruisanchez, C, Dawson, D, Grapsa, J, North, B, Howard, L.S, Pinto, F.J, Nihoyannopoulos, P, & Gibbs, J.R.S. Right ventricular function in patients with pulmonary hypertension; the value of myocardial performance index measured by tissue Doppler imaging. Eur J Echocardiogr. (2010)., 11(8), 719-724.

[54] Miller, D, Farah, M.G, Liner, A, Fox, K, Schluchter, M, & Hoit, B.D. The relation between quantitative right ventricular ejection fraction and indices of tricuspid annular motion and myocardial perfromance. J Am Soc Echocardiogr. (2004)., 17(5), 443-447.

[55] Forfia, P.R, Fisher, M.R, Mathai, S.C, Housten-Harris, T, Hemnes, A.R, Borlaug, B.A, Chamera, E, Corretti, E, Champion, H.C, Abraham, T.P, Girgis R.E, & Hassoun, P.M. Tricuspid annular displacement predicts survival in pulmonary hypertension. Am J Respir Crit Care Med. (2006)., 174(9), 1034-1041.

[56] Kaul, S, Tei, C, Hopkins, J.M, & Shah, P.M. Assessment of right ventricular function using two-dimensional echocardiography. Am Heart J. (1984)., 107(3), 526-531.

[57] Lindqvist, P, Waldenstrom, A, Henein, M, Morner, S, & Kazzam, E. Regional and global right ventricular function in normal individuals aged 20-90 years: a pulsed Doppler tissue imaging study: Umea General Population Heart Study. Echocardiogr. (2005)., 22(4), 305-314.

[58] Lindqvist, P, Waldenstrom, A, Wikstrom, G, & Kazzam, E. The use of isovolumic contraction velocity to determine right ventricular state of contractility and filling

pressures: A pulsed Doppler tissue imaging study. Eur J Echocardiogr. (2005)., 6(4), 264-270.

[59] Kukulski, N.P, Hubbert, L, Arnold, M, Wranne, B, Hatle, L, & Sutherland, G.R. Normal regional right ventricular function and its change with age: a Doppler myocardial imaging study. J Am Soc Echocardiogr. (2000)., 13(3), 194-204.

[60] Bleeker, G.B, Steendijk, P, Holman, E.R, Yu, C.M, Breitharth, O.A, Kaandorp, T.A.M, Schalij, M.J, van der Wall, E.E, Nihoyannopoulos, P, & Bax, J.J. Assessing right ventricular function: the role of echocardiography and complementary technologies. Heart. (2006)., 92(Suppl 1), i19–i26.

[61] Vogel, M, Schmidt, M.R, Kristiansen, S.B, Cheung, M, White, P.A, Sorensen, K, & Redington, A.N. Validation of myocardial acceleration during isovolumic contraction as a novel noninvasive index of right ventricular contractility: comparison with ventricular pressure-volume relations in an animal model. Circulation. (2002)., 105(14), 1693-1699.

[62] Hashimoto, I, Li, X.K, Hejmadi Bhat, A, Jones, M, & Sahn, D.J. Quantitative assessment of regional peak myocardial acceleration during isovolumic contraction and relaxation time by tissue Doppler imaging. Heart. (2005)., 91(6), 811-816.

[63] Tayyareci, Y, Tayyareci, G, Tastan, C.P, Bayazit, P, & Nisanci, Y. Early diagnosis of right ventricular systolic dysfunction by tissue Doppler-derived isovolumic myocardial acceleration in patients with chronic obstructive pulmonary disease. Echocardiogr. (2009)., 26(9), 1026-1035.

[64] Tugcu, A, Yildirimturk, O, Tayyareci, Y, Demiroglu, C, & Aytekin, S. Evaluation of subclinical right ventricular dysfunction in obstructive sleep apnea patients using velocity vector imaging. Circ J. (2010)., 74(2), 312-319.

[65] Tayyareci, Y, Yurdakul, S, Tayyareci, G, Nisanci, Y, Umman, B, & Bugra, Z. Impact of myocardial acceleration during isovolumic contraction in evaluating subclinical right ventricular systolic dysfunction in type 2 diabetes mellitus patients. Echocardiogr. (2010)., 27(10), 1211-1218.

[66] Tayyareci, Y, Nisanci, Y, Umman, B, Oncul, A, Yurdakul, S, Altun, I, Umman, S, & Bugra, Z. Early detection of right ventricular systolic dysfunction by using myocardial acceleration during isovolumic contraction in patients with mitral stenosis. Eur J Echocardiogr. (2008)., 9(4), 516-521.

[67] Schattke, S, Knebel, F, Grohmann, A, Dreger, H, Kmezik, F, Riemekasten, G, Baumann, G, & Borges, A.C. Early right ventricular systolic dysfunction in patients with systemic sclerosis without pulmonary hypertension: a Doppler Tissue and Speckle Tracking echocardiography study. Cardiovasc Ultrasound. (2010)., 8, 3.

[68] Arnold, R, Gorenflo, M, Böttler, P, Eichhorn, J, Jung, C, & Goebel, B. Tissue Doppler derived isovolumic acceleration in patients after atrial repair for dextrotransposition of the great arteries. Echocardiogr. (2008)., 25(7), 732-738.

[69] Nikitin, N.P, Loh, P.H, De Silva, R, Witte, K.K, Lukaschuk, E.I, Parker, A, Farnsworth, T.A, Alamgir, F.M, Clark, A.L, & Cleland, J.G. Left ventricular morphology, global and longitudinal function in normal older individuals: a cardiac magnetic resonance study. Int J Cardiol. (2006)., 108(1), 76-83.

[70] Dalen, H, Thorstensen, A, Vatten, L.J, Aase, S.A, & Stoylen, A. Reference Values and Distribution of Conventional Echocardiographic Doppler Measures and Longitudinal Tissue Doppler Velocities in a Population Free From Cardiovascular Disease. Circ Cardiovasc Imaging. (2010)., 3(5), 614-622.

[71] Meluzin, J, Spinarova, L, Bakala, J, Toman, J, Hude, P, Kara, T, & Soucek, M. Pulsed Doppler tissue imaging of the velocity of tricuspid annular systolic motion. A new, rapid, and non-invasive method of evaluating right ventricular systolic function. Eur Heart J. (2001)., 22(4), 340-348.

[72] Lopez-Candales, A, Dohi, K, Bazaz, R, & Edelman, K. Relation of right ventricular free wall mechanical delay to right ventricular dysfunction as determined by tissue Doppler imaging. Am J Cardiol. (2005)., 96(4), 602-606.

[73] Rojo, E.C, Rodrigo, J.L, Perez de Isla, R, Almeria, C, Gonzalo, N, Aubele, A, Cinza, R, Zamorano, J, & Macaya, C. Disagreement between tissue Doppler imaging and conventional pulsed wave Doppler in the measurement of myocardial performance index. Eur J Echocardiogr. (2006)., 7(5), 356-364.

[74] Gaibazzi, N, Petrucci, N, & Ziacchi, V. Left ventricle myocardial performance index derived either by conventional method or mitral annulus tissue Doppler: a comparison study in healthy subjects and subjects with heart failure. J Am Soc Echocardiogr. (2005)., 18(12), 1270-1276.

[75] Duzenli, M.A, Ozdemir, K, Aygul, N, Soylu, A, Aygul, M.U, & Gok, H. Comparison of myocardial performance index obtained either by conventional echocardiography or tissue Doppler echocardiography in healthy subjects and patients with heart failure. Heart Vessels. (2009)., 24(1), 8-15.

[76] Abd El Rahman, M.Y, Hui, W, Dsebissowa, F, Schubert, S, Hubler, M, Hetzer, R, Lange, P.E, & Abdul-Kahliq, H. Comparison of the tissue Doppler-derived left ventricular Tei index to than obtained by Doppler in patients with congenital and acquired hear disease. Pediatr Cardiol. (2005)., 26(4),391-395.

[77] Chockalingam, A, Gnanavelu, G, Alagesan, R, & Subramaniam, T. Myocardial performance index in evaluation of acute right ventricular myocardial infarction. Echocardiogr. (2004)., 21(6), 487-494.

[78] Blanchard, D.G, Malouf, P.J, Gurudevan, S.V, Auger, V.R, Madani, M.M, Thistlethwhite, P, Waltman, T.J, Daniels, L.B, Raisinghani, A.B, DeMaria, A.N. Utility of right

ventricular Tei indexin the noninvasive evaluation of chronic thromboembolic pulmonary hypertension before and after pulmonary thromboendarterectomy. JACC Cardiovasc Imaging. (2009)., 2(2),143-149.

[79] Hsiao, S.H, Lee, C.Y, Chang, S.M, Yang, S.H, Lin, S.K, & Huang, W.C. Pulmonary embolism and right heart function: insights from myocardial Doppler tissue imaging. J Am Soc Echocardiogr. (2006)., 19(6), 822-828.

[80] Hsiao, S.H, Yang, S.H, Wang, W.C, Lee, C.Y, Lin, S.K, & Liu, C.P. Usefulness of regional myocardial performance index to diagnose pulmonary embolism in patients with echocardiographic signs of pulmonary hypertension. Am J Cardiol. (2006)., 98(12), 1652-1655.

[81] Park, J.H, Park, Y.S, Park, S.J, Lee, J.H, Choi, S.W, Jeong, J.O, & Seong, I.W. Midventricular peak systolic strain and Tei index of the right ventricle correlated with decreased right ventricular systolic function in patients with acute pulmonary thromboembolism. Int J Cardiol. (2006)., 125(3), 319-324.

[82] Haddad, F, Denault, A.Y, Couture, P, Cartier, R, Pellerin, M, Levesque, S, Lambert, J, & Tardif, J.C. Right ventricular myocardial performance index predicts perioperative mortality or circulatory failure in high-risk valvular surgery. J Am Soc Echocardiogr. (2007)., 20(9), 1065-1072.

[83] Ishii, M, Eto, G, Tei, C, Tsutsumi, T, Hashino, K, Sugahara, Y, Himeno, W, Muta, H, Furui, J, Akagi, T, Fukiyama, R, Toyoda, O, & Kato, H. Quantitation of the global right ventricular function in children with normal heart and congenital heart disease: a right ventricular myocardial performance index. Pediatr Cardiol. (2000)., 21(5), 416-421.

[84] Eidem, B.W, Tei, C, O'Leary, P.W, Cetta, F, & Seward, J.B. No geometric quantitative assessment of right and left ventricular function: Myocardial performance index in normal children and patients with Ebstein anomaly. J Am Soc Echocardiogr. (1998)., 11(9), 849-856.

[85] Romero-Corral, A, Somers, V.K, Pellikka, P.A, Olson, E.J, Bailey, K.R, Korinek, J, Orban, M, Sierra-Johnson, J, Kato, M, Amin, R.S, & Lopez-Jimenez, F. Decreased Right and Left Ventricular Myocardial Performance in Obstructive Sleep Apnea. Chest. (2007)., 132(6), 1863-1870.

[86] Jurcut, R, Giusca, S, La Gerche, A, Vasile, S, Ginghina, C, & Voigt, J.U. The echocardiographic assessment of the right ventricle: what to do in 2010? Eur J Echocardiogr. (2010)., 11(2), 81-96.

[87] Brecker, S.J.D, Gibbs, J.S.G, Fox, K.M, Yacoub, M.H, & Gibson, D.G. Comparison of Doppler derived haemodynamic variables and simultaneous high fidelity pressure measurements in severe pulmonary hypertension. Br Heart J. (1994)., 72(4), 384-389.

[88] Anconina, J, Danchin, N, Selton-Suty, C, Isaaz, K, Juilliere, Y, Buffet, P, Edel, F, & Cherrier, F. Measurement of right ventricular dp/dt. A simultaneous/comparative he-

modynamic and Doppler echocardiographic study. Arch Mal Coeur Vaiss. (1992)., 85(9), 1317-1321.

[89] Kanzaki, H, Nakatani, S, Kawada, T, Yamagishi, M, Sunagawa, K, & Miyatake, K. Right ventricular dP/dt/P(max), not dP/dt(max), noninvasively derived from tricuspid regurgitation velocity is a useful index of right ventricular contractility. J Am Soc Echocardiogr. (2002)., 15(2), 136-142.

[90] Galie, N, Hoeper, M.M, Humbert, M, Torbicki, A, Vachiery, J.L, Barbera, J.A, Beghetti, M, Corris, P, Gaine, S, Gibbs, J.S, Gomes-Sanchez, M.A, Jondeau, G, Klepetko, W, Opitz, C, Rubin, L, Zellweger, M, & Simonneau, G. Guidelines for the diagnostis and treatment of pulmonary artery hypertension. Eur Heart J. (2009)., 30(20), 2493-2537.

[91] Habib, G, & Torbiki, A. The role of echocardiography in the diagnosis and management of patients with pulmonary hypertension. Eur Respir Rev. (2010)., 19(118), 288-299.

[92] Abraham, J, & Abraham, T.P. The Role of Echocardiography in Hemodinamic Assessment in Heart failure. Heart Fail Clin. (2009)., 5(2), 191-208.

[93] Ristow, B, & Schiller, N.B. Stepping away from ritual right heart catheterisation into the era of non-invasively measured pulmonary artery pressure. J Am Soc Echocardiogr. (2009)., 22(7), 820-822.

[94] Milan, A, Magnino, C, & Veglio, C. Echocardiographic indexes for the non-invasive evaluation of pulmonary hemodynamics. J Am Soc Echocardiogr. (2010)., 23(3), 225-239.

[95] Dabestani, A, Mahan, G, Gardin, JM, Takenaka, K, Burn, C, Allfie, A, & Henry, W.L. Evaluation of the pulmonary artery pressure and resistance by Doppler echocardiography. Am J Cardiol. (1987)., 59 (6), 662-668.

[96] Fisher, M.R, Forfia, F.R, Chamera, E, Housten-Harris, T, Champion, H.C, Girgis, R.E, Corretti, M.C, & Hassoun, P.M. Accuracy of Echocardiography in the hemodynamic assessment of pulmonary hypertension. Am J Respir Crit Care Med. (2009)., 179(7), 615-621.

[97] McGoon, M, Gutterman, D, Steen, V, Barst, R, McCrory, D.C, Fortin, T.A, & Loyd, J.E. Screening, early detection and diagnosis of pulmonary arterial hypertension: ACCP evidence-based clinical practice guidelines. Chest. (2004)., 126(suppl 1), 14S-34S.

[98] Ozdemir, K, Altunkeser, B.B, Icli, A, Ozdil, H, & Gok, H. New Parameters in identification of right ventricle myocardial infarction and proximal right coronary artery lesion. Chest. (2003)., 124(1), 219-226.

[99] Kowalski, M, Kukulski, T, Jamal, F, D'hooge, J, Weidemann, F, Rademakers, F, Bijnens, B, Hatle, L, & Sutherland, G.R. Can natural strain and strain rate quantify re-

gional myocardial deformation? A study in healthy subjects. Ultrasound Med Biol. (2001)., 27(8), 1087-1097.

[100] Marwick TH. Measurement of strain and strain rate by echocardiography: ready for prime time? J Am Coll Cardiol. (2006)., 47(7), 1313-1327.

[101] Teske, A.J, De Boeck, B.W, Olimulder, M, Prakken, N.H, Doevendans, P.A, & Cramer, M.J. Echocardiographic assessment of regional right ventricular function: a head-to-head comparison between 2-dimensional and tissue Doppler-derived strain analysis. J Am Soc Echocardiogr. (2008)., 21(3), 275-283.

[102] Cho, E.J, Jiamsripong, P, Calleja, A.M, Alharthi, M.S, McMahon, E.M, Khandheria, B.K, & Belohlavek, M. Right ventricular free wall circumferential strain reflects graded elevation in acute right ventricular afterload. Am J Physiol Heart Circ Physi. (2009)., 296(2), H413-H420.

[103] Benza, R, Biederman, R, Murali, S, & Gupta, H. Role of cardiac magnetic resonance imaging in the management of patients with pulmonary arterial hypertension. J Am Coll Cardiol. 2008; 52(21):1683-1692.

[104] Maceira, A.M, Prasad, S.K, Khan, M, & Pennell, D.J. Reference right ventricular systolic and diastolic function normalized to age, gender and body surface area from steady-state free precession cardiovascular magnetic resonance. Eur Heart J. (2006)., 27(23), 2879-2888.

[105] Leibundgut, G, Rohner, A, Grize, L, Bernheim, A, Kessel-Schaefer, A, Bremerich, J, Zellweger, M, Buser, P, & Handke, M. Dynamic Assessment of Right Ventricular Volumes and Function by Real-Time Three-Dimensional Echocardiography: A Comparison Study With Magnetic Resonance Imaging in 100 Adult Patients. J Am Soc Echocardiogr. (2010)., 23(2), 116-126.

[106] Lu, X, Nadvoretskiy, V, Bu, L, Stolpen, A, Ayres, N, Pignatelli, R.H, Kovalchin, J.P, Grenier, M, Klas, B, & Ge, S. Accuracy and reproducibility of real-time three-dimensional echocardiography for assessment of right ventricular volumes and ejection fraction in children. J Am Soc Echocardiogr. (2008)., 21(1), 84-89.

[107] Kjaergaard, J, Petersen, C.L, Kjaer, A, Schaadt, BK, Oh, J.K, & Hassager, C. Evaluation of right ventricular volume and function by 2D and 3D echocardiography compared to MRI. Eur J Echocardiogr. (2006)., 7(6), 430-438.

[108] Vonk-Noordegraaf, A, Marcus, J.T, Gan, C.T, Boonstra, A, & Postmus, P.E. Interventricular mechanical asynchrony due to right ventricular pres-sure overload in pulmonary hypertension plays an important role in impaired left ventricular filling. Chest. (2005)., 128(Suppl 6), 628S–630S.

[109] Crean, A.M, Maredia, N, Ballard, G, Menezes, R, Wharton, G, Forster, J, Greenwood, J.P, & Thomson, J.D. 3D Echo systematically underestimates right ventricular volumes compared to cardiovascular magnetic resonance in adult congenital heart dis-

ease patients with moderate or severe RV dilatation. J Cardiovasc Magn Reson. (2011)., 13, 78.

[110] Wang, J, Prakasa, K, Bomma, C, Tandri, H, Dalal, D, James, C, Tichnell, C, Corretti, M, Bluemke, D, Calkins, H, & Abraham, T.P. Comparison of novel echocardiographic parameters of right ventricular function with ejection fraction by cardiac magnetic resonance. J Am Soc Echocardiogr. (2007)., 20(9), 1058-1064.

[111] Pavlicek, M, Wahl, A, Rutz, T, De Marchi, S.F, Hille, R, Wustmann, K, Steck, H, Eigenmann, C, Schwerzmann, M, & Seiler, C. Right ventricular systolic function assessment: rank of echocardiographic methods vs. cardiac magnetic resonance imaging. Eur J Echocardiogr. (2011)., 12(11), 871-880.

[112] Klein, A.L, Leung, D.Y, Murray, R.D, Urban, L.H, Bailey, K.R, & Tajik, A.J. Effects of age and physiologic variables on right ventricular filling dynamics in normal subjects. Am J Cardiol. (1999)., 84(4), 440-448.

[113] Berman, J.L, Green, L.H, & Grossman, W. Right ventricular diastolic pressure in coronary artery disease. Chest. (1979)., 44(7), 1263-1268.

[114] Marwick TH. Clinical application of tissue Doppler imaging: a promise fulfilled. Heart. (2003)., 89(12), 1377-1378.

[115] Pellerin, D, Sharma, R, Elliot, P, & Veyrat, C. Tissue Doppler, strain, and strain rate echocardiography for the assessment of left and right systolic ventricular function. Heart. (2003)., 89(suppl 3), iii9-17.

[116] Yu, C.M, Lin, H, Ho, P.C, & Yang, H. Assessment of left and right ventricular systolic and diastolic synchronicity in normal subjects by tissue Doppler echocardiography and the effects of age and heart rate. Echocardiography. (2003)., 20(1), 19-27.

[117] Yalcin, F, Kaftan, A, Muderrisoglu, H, Korkmaz, M.E, Flachskampf, F, Garcia, M, & Thomas, J.D. Is Doppler tissue velocity during early left ventricular filling preload independent? Heart. (2002)., 87 (4), 336-339.

[118] Pela, G, Regolisti, G, Coghi, P, Cabassi, A, Basile, A, Cavatorta, A, Manca, C, & Borghetti, A. Effects of the reduction of preload on left and right myocardial velocities analysed by Doppler tissue echocardiography in healthy subjects. Eur J Echocardiogr. (2004)., 5(4), 262-271.

[119] Horton, K.D, Meece, R.W, & Hill, J.C. Assessment of the right ventricle by echocardiography: a primer for cardiac sonographers. J Am Soc Echocardiogr. (2009)., 22(7), 776-792.

[120] Puwanat, S, Priester, T.C, Mookadam, F, Bruce, C.J, Redfield, M.M, & Chandrasekaran, K. Right ventricular function in patients with heart failure and preserved ejection fraction. Eur J Echocardiogr. (2009)., 10(6), 733-737.

[121] Utsunomiya, H, Nakatani, S, Nishihira, M, Kanzaki, H, Kyotani, S, Nakanishi, N, Kihara, Y, & Kitakaze, M. Value of Estimated Right Ventricular Filling Pressure in Pre-

dicting Cardiac Events in Chronic Pulmonary Arterial Hypertension. J Am Soc Echocardiogr. (2009)., 22(12), 1368-1374.

[122] Kayser, H.W, van der Geest, R.J, van der Wall, E.E, Duchateau, C, & De Roos, A. Right ventricular function in patients after acute myocardial infarction assessed with phase contrast MR velocity mapping encoded in three directions. J Magn Reson Imaging. (2000)., 11(5), 471-475.

[123] Paelinck, B.P, De Roos, A, Bax, J.J, Bosmans, J.M, van der Geest, R.J, Dhondt, D, Parizel, P.M, Vrints, C.J, & Lamb, H.J. Feasibility of tissue magnetic resonance imaging: a pilot study in comparison with tissue Doppler imaging and invasive measurement. J Am Coll Cardiol. (2005)., 45(7), 1109-1116.

[124] Janda, S, Shahidi, N, Gin, K, & Swiston, J. Diagnostic accuracy of echocardiography for pulmonary hypertension: a systematic review and meta-analysis. Heart. (2011)., 97(8), 612-622.

[125] Sitbon, O, Humbert, M, Jais, X, Ioos, V, Hamid, A.M, Provencher, S, Garcia, G, Parent, F, Herve, P, & Simonneau, G. Long-term response to calcium channel blockers in idiopathic pulmonary arterial hypertension. Circulation. (2005)., 111(23), 3105–3111.

Chapter 3

Lung Ultrasound Comet Tails — Technique and Clinical Significance

Douglas T. Summerfield and Bruce D. Johnson

Additional information is available at the end of the chapter

http://dx.doi.org/10.5772/56198

1. Introduction

While often overlooked by traditional echocardiography, the lungs and evaluation of extravascular lung water (EVLW) can be assessed by direct visualization with relatively simple ultrasonographic techniques. The results can help guide clinicians towards the cause of a patient's dyspnea and in the case of pulmonary edema even semi-quantitatively asses EVLW. Additionally the exam can be repeated as often as necessary to monitor response to treatment without fear of subjecting the patient to ionizing radiation associated with conventional chest radiography.

Advancing technology has allowed for increasingly miniaturized and portable ultrasound systems to the point where exams can be performed quickly at the bedside, often by the rounding physician. The more common standard of care for quantifying pulmonary edema has been a chest radiograph which, depending on the institution, may require more time to perform and a more formal interpretation than a portable ultrasound [1]. Even when it is obtained, chest radiograph can have a low sensitivity for common causes of dyspnea such as pulmonary edema [2, 3]. This may be due in part to poor radiographic windows of the patient or the intraobserver variability and skills of those interpreting the x-ray [4, 5]. In the case of acute pulmonary edema, the practitioner using techniques of lung ultrasound, can actually visualize the edema, classify it semi-quantitatively, and prescribe interventions before other traditional diagnostic techniques such as chest radiograph can even occur.

The lung ultrasound finding of "Comet Tails" has been well studied in how it relates to alveolar-interstitial syndromes. These syndromes include conditions with diffuse involvement of the pulmonary interstitium which lead to respiratory distress through impairment of alveolar-capillary exchange. Chronic conditions include pulmonary fibrosis, whereas acute entities are acute respiratory distress syndrome (ARDS), interstitial pneumonia, and acute pulmonary edema [5]. With careful attention paid by the examiner at the bedside to the patient's history and monitoring the response to treatment, the ultrasonographic finding of comet tails can be extremely useful in narrowing the differential diagnosis.

2. Definitions

"A-lines and B-lines" are two separate and distinct ultrasonographic images which may be seen during examination of the lungs by ultrasound (See Figures 1 &2). Their presence is not mutually exclusive, but the formation of each arises from a different underlying structure.

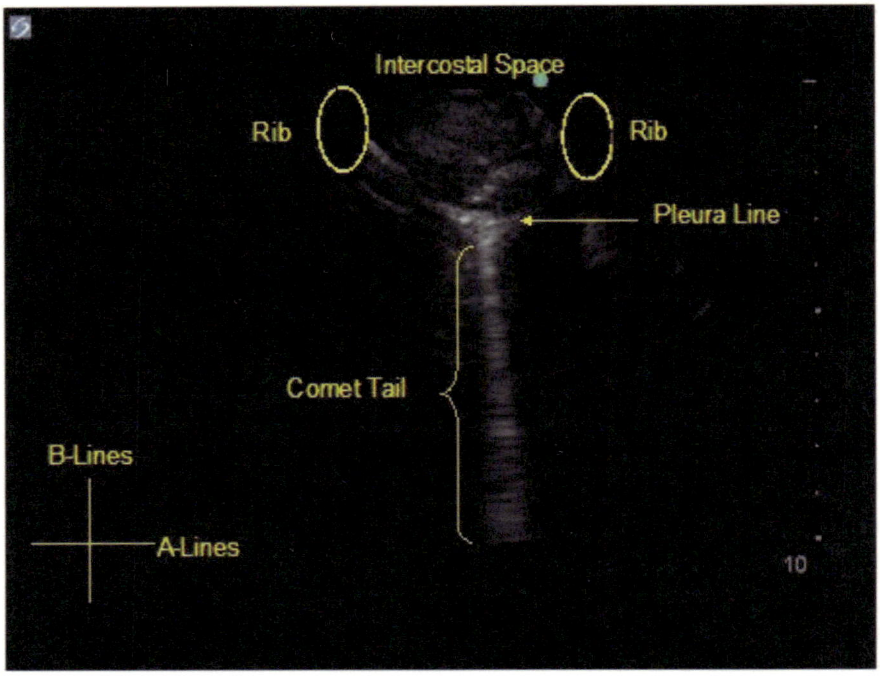

Figure 1. Image of comet tail "B-lines"

Comet-tails or "B-lines" are defined as hyperechoic reflections which originate only from and travel roughly perpendicular to the pleural line of the lung. They have a narrow base and form a ray spreading away from the transducer towards the bottom of the screen and synchronously move with lung respiration. All ultrasound images are formed when a reflection occurs at the interface of two regions with differing acoustic impedance [6]. In the case of comet tails this impedance occurs between fluid filled interlobular septa, with the acoustic impedance of water being $1.48x10^5gp/cm^2$ and that of an air filled lung with the acoustic impedance of air being of $0.0004x10^5gp/cm^2$. Interlobular septa are structures within the lung containing lymphatic vessels. These septa are below the resolution of the ultrasound beam, which can only detect

http://dx.doi.org/10.5772/56198

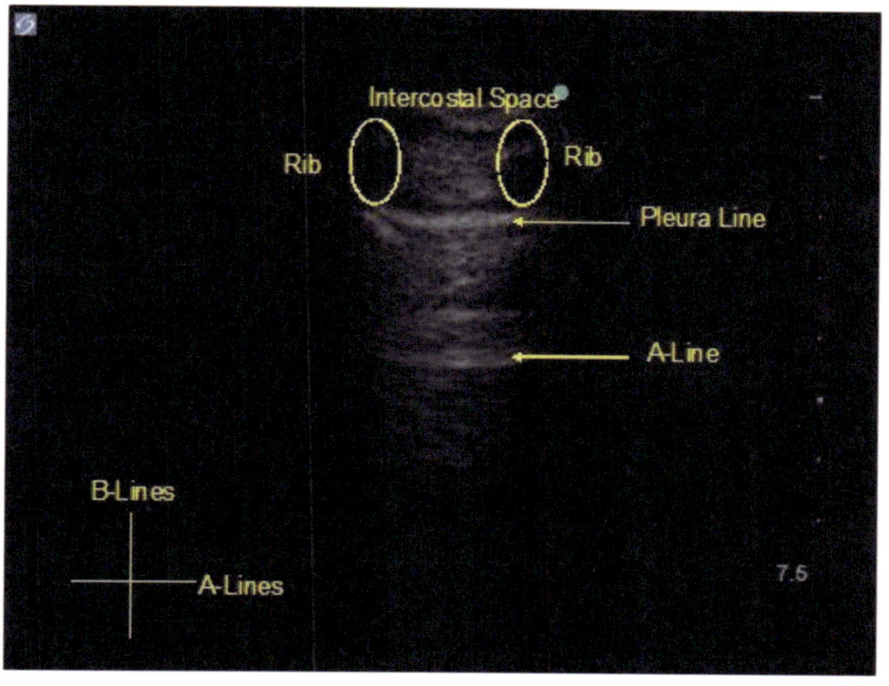

Figure 2. Image of pleural "A-lines."

objects larger than 1 mm. Instead of showing up as a distinct structure, in the right circumstances the areas of highly different acoustic impedance show up as a comet tail [7,8].

Under normal (non-edematous or fibrotic) conditions comet tails are absent because no acoustic mismatch occurs as the beam passes through the subpleural space. However, in conditions known as alveolar-interstitial syndromes an area of high acoustic mismatch occurs at the subpleural space were interlobular septa are in contact with the pleural lining. In the case of pulmonary edema this mismatch occurs between the differing impedances of air and water, however it can also occur anytime there is an area of differing impedances at the surface of the lungs such as pleuritis, fibrosis, or even chronic obstructive pulmonary disease [9].

Even though these structures are smaller than the resolution of the ultrasound beam, the reflections cans still be generated and sent back to the ultrasound probe. Continued reflections set up the phenomenon of reverberation which acts as a continued source of reflections back to the piezoelectric crystal. Since the ultrasound interprets time as distance, and each successive echo or return to the transducer occurs over a more distant time than the original signal, the ultrasound interprets these signals as reflections from a structure more distal from the ultrasound probe [6]. In this way a "beam" or comet tail image is created on the echo screen. (See Figure 3) Histologically the interlobular septa are 7 mm apart when they reach the sub pleural space and this is roughly the distance between the origins of individual comet tails at the pleural line [7].

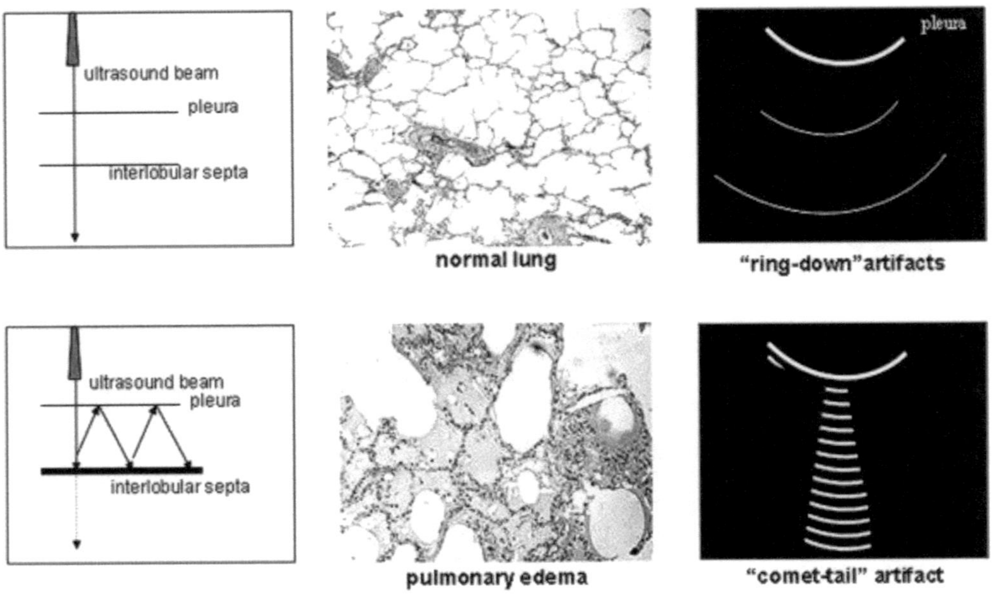

Figure 3. The hypothesized physical and anatomic basis of echocardiographic lung comet tails. Reflections of the ultrasound beam between thickened interlobular septa and the pleura generate a resonance signal over a prolonged time. The increased return over time is interpreted by the ultrasound machine as a hyperechoic structure originating deeper in the tissue and is displayed as a comet-tail on the ultrasound screen. (Illustrations and images from Jambrik et al. Usefulness of ultrasound lung comets as a nonradiologic sign of extravascular lung water. Am J Cardiol 2004;93:1265-1270, with permission from Excerpta Medica, Inc.)

For the comet tail image to form, these thickened intralobular septa must be in contact with the sub pleural space as any air between them and the transducer has such a low acoustic impedance that the echo return takes too long and is simply "cancelled out" by the machine. (This is the reason lung comets are not seen in pneumothorax and can aid in the diagnosis of that condition.) [6] In a traditional chest radiograph these septa thickened by pulmonary edema are termed "Kerley B-lines" [10, 11].

A-Lines are another distinct ultrasonographic entity separate from the "B-line" comet tails. A-lines are hyperechoic lines which run roughly horizontal across the ultrasound screen and are parallel to the pleural line. These lines are equidistant to each other and are the same distance from each other as the pleural line is from the skin because they are reverberations of the pleural line. Again the ultrasound machine interprets the signals it receives temporally from the reverberations as depth. Hence the reflections are seen as lines deeper on the screen. The presence of A-lines, and absence of B-lines indicates the presence of "dry" intralobular septa and is a strong predictor of a normal capillary wedge pressure [12].

http://dx.doi.org/10.5772/56198

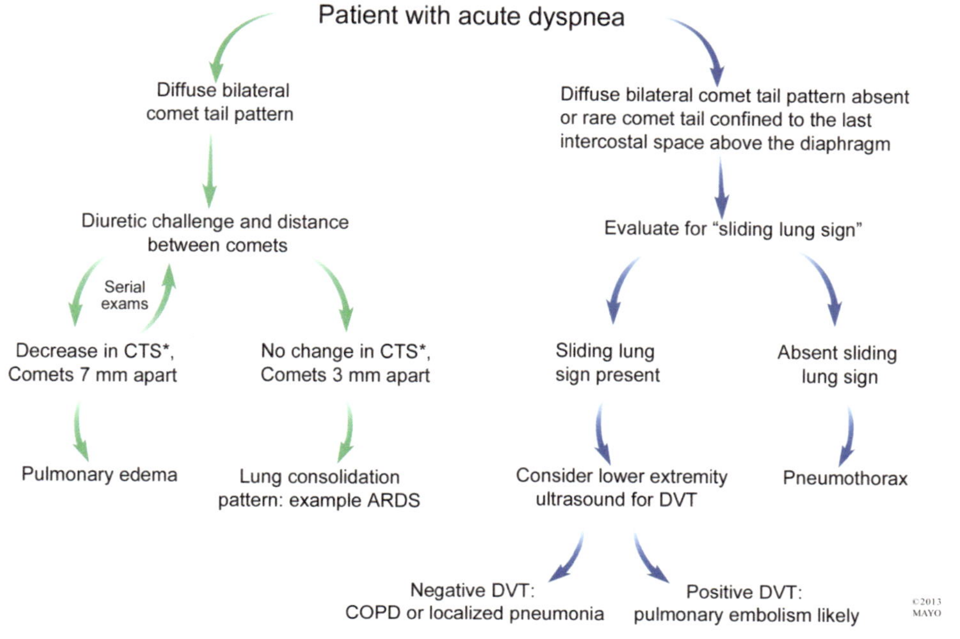

*CTS: Comet Tail Score.

Figure 4. Proposed algorithm for use of lung comet tails in the evaluation of patients with acute dyspnea. In the case of pulmonary edema, serial ultrasonographic exams performed after therapeutic intervention(s) will reveal a diminishing number of comet tails. This algorithm is suggested as a possible supplement for typical clinical assessment in the decision making process.

3. History and origins

The "comet-tail" ultrasonographic sign was first described by Ziskin and colleagues in 1982 when an intrahepatic shotgun pellet was observed to create an artifact similar to what is seen in lung comets [8]. Other conditions affecting the pleura of the lung were later noted to create a similar pattern [9]. However it was not until 1997 when Daniel Lichtenstein, a French critical care physician, described lung comet tails as an ultrasonographic sign of alveolar-interstitial syndrome. In his paper he examined 250 patients, 121 with evidence of either wide-spread (N=92) or localized (N=29) evidence of alveolar-interstitial syndrome on chest x-ray and 129 patients with a normal chest radiograph. He found the sensitivity of ultrasound in detecting this pattern was 93.4% with a specificity of 93.0% in patients who did not have evidence for this on chest x-ray [7].

When Lichtenstein compared chest computerized tomography (CT) to the ultrasound findings on 29 of his 250 patients, he found comet tails were generated diffusely across the lungs from two distinct sources. Both of these sources were lesions associated with acute pulmonary edema, thickened sub-pleural interlobular septa and ground-glass regions. Occasionally even "normal" subjects registered the rare comet tail in the diaphragmatic regions of the lung, and this was detected in both x-ray and CT scan [7].

Clinical applications of comet tails began after Jambrik and colleagues evaluated 121 hospitalized patients with lung ultrasound (see technique below) and compared the findings to chest x-ray. They found a significant linear correlation between a comet tail score (CTS) and x-ray ($r=0.78$, $p<.01$). When patients were examined multiple times, an even higher intrapatient correlation was seen ($r=0.89$; $p<0.01$). [13]

Lichtenstein and Jambrik's observations were expanded to the medical in-patient setting by Tsereva who validated the technique in patients with diastolic heart failure [14] and by Volpicelli, who validated the use of ultrasound in diagnosis alveolar interstitial syndrome with a 85.7% sensitivity and 97.7% specificity. The lower sensitivity in the later study can be explained by the timing of the x-ray and the ultrasounds. The chest radiographs which the ultrasounds were compared to were taken at admission and guided the treatment given, whereas the lung ultrasounds were done after the initiation of therapy. Thus for some patients the lack of comet tails was merely the resolution of pulmonary edema, but in the analysis resulted in a lower sensitivity of the ultrasound technique [5]. Other researchers further validated lung ultrasound and have suggested that it is superior to chest x-ray with sensitivities similar to Nt-proBNP levels [15]. Nt-proBNP (N-terminal probrain type natriuretic peptide) has become a common biomarker for fluid overload and tracking health status in heart failure patients. However, fluid overload may not always correlate with interstitial pulmonary edema and thus may be a marker primarily of vascular fluid overload.

In an effort to help quantify the number of comet tails seen on exam, Agricola et al. evaluated post-cardiac surgery patients. They devised a relatively simple definition for a positive or negative comet tail exam. A positive comet tail test was simply multiple bilateral comet tails seen over the whole lung surface. A negative test was with the rare occasional comet tail, the absence of comet tails, or comet tails confined to the last intercostals space. They then compared the patient's comet tail test to the amount of extravascular lung water (EVLW) determined by Pulse Contour Cardiac Output (PiCCO - is an invasive technique requiring catheters and uses principals of transpulmonary thermodilution and arterial pulse contour analysis in order to estimate extravascular lung water), to the patient's wedge pressure, and to their radiologic score as determined by chest x-ray. Again good correlation was seen between the radiologic assessment of EVLW and comet tails ($r=0.60$, $p<0.0001$) and also when compared to wedge pressure ($r=0.48$, $p<0.0001$). Most useful was the comparison to EVLW. Normal EVLW is <500 mL with alveolar flooding occurring when EVLW reaches more than 75% above its normal limit [16, 17]. With this in mind, the negative test had a 90% sensitivity and 89% specificity of accurately detecting an EVLW volume <500 mL. Likewise a positive test had a 90% and 86% sensitivity and specificity of detecting EVLW >500 mL. When comparing the comet tail test to chest radiographs and PiCCO, they found they were even able to detect excess EVLW below the threshold which would cause alveolar edema (sub clinical or early stages of pulmonary edema) with 87% and 89% sensitivity and specificity [11].

Monitoring EVLW through the formation of lung comet tails was shown to be even more important than knowing a patients overall volume status. Using bioelectric impedance

Mallamaci demonstrated that in dialysis patients, overall volume status was not linked to pulmonary congestion and the formation of comet tails. Rather Comet tails, and pulmonary congestion, had more to do with a patient's left ventricular function. They also demonstrated the ability of comet tails to detect patient who were asymptomatic as 57% of patients had moderate to severe pulmonary congestion but did not have symptoms suggesting such [18]. This is in keeping with Lichtenstein's original paper which discussed a patient with a fat embolism who had the sonographic sign of comet tails three days before symptoms occurred [7] and in older literature which argued that alveolar edema, which would lead to symptoms, is preceded by interstitial edema (which may or may not cause symptoms but can now be detected by ultrasound) [19].

4. Technique

The standard technique for quantification of comet tails has been reported in a number of studies and was pioneered by Picano and colleagues [9,13, 11]. This technique has shown its utility clinically as used by the Himalayan Rescue Association to help diagnose and monitor the degree of pulmonary edema in high-altitude pulmonary edema (HAPE). [20]

The exam is performed using any commercially available portable ultrasound device which has a 1-7 MHz phased array probe. We recommend the use of the 1-5 MHz cardiac probe as it is ideal for viewing between rib spaces and still allows deep enough penetration of the ultrasound beam to view distal structures. Other groups have also found adequate views with the high frequency linear probes as well as the abdominal probes as well [21].

The patient is placed in a supine or near supine position with the anterior chest wall exposed. Each intercostals space from the second to the fifth on the right and the second to the fourth on the left is scanned in four different positions. These are para-sternal, midclavicular, anterior axillary, and mid-axillary. This gives the examiner a total of 28 different windows to examine, 16 on the right and 12 on the left (See graphic representation Table 1).

Right Hemithorax					Left Hemithorax			
Mid-Axillary	Anterior axillary	Mid-clavicular	Para-Sternal	Inter-costal space	Para-Sternal	Mid-clavicular	Anterior axillary	Mid-axillary

Table 1. Diagram of the ultrasound windows used to obtain the Comet Tail Score (CTS). This technique was proposed by Jambrik at al. and used by Jambrik, Fagenholtz, Pratali, Agricola, Picano, Mallamaci. Each window is evaluated for comet tails, and the number present is added to form a cumulative score.

Within each window, comet tails as defined above are counted. The sum of the comet tails seen can then be compiled for a comet tail score (CTS). The intra- and interobserver variability using this method has been reported as 5.1% and 7.4% respectively [13]. For clinical purposes Picano and colleges report the comet tail score in a semiquantitative manner for patients in pulmonary edema (Table 2).

Score	Number of Comet Tails	EVLW
0	<5	No Signs
1	5-15	Mild
2	15-30	Moderate
3	"/>30	Severe

Table 2. Semiquantitive classification of the Comet Tail Score (CTS)as proposed by Picano and colleagues.

4.1. Other techniques

Simpler less quantitative techniques have also been described with good prediction of pulmonary edema. Volpicelli and colleagues described a technique where each hemithorax is divided into four quadrants (8 total), upper and lower anterior and upper and lower lateral divided longitudinally by the anterior axillary line and transversely by the 2nd intercostal space. An exam was considered abnormal (positive for edema) if it had all of the following features:

1. At least three comet tails per scan.
2. Diffusely positive with more than one scan per side containing comet tails.
3. Bilateral presence of comet tails.

By using these criteria this group found a 85.7% sensitivity and 97.7% specificity when compared to chest x-ray for detecting the presence of pulmonary edema [5].

5. Application and differential diagnosis

The presence of occasional sporadic comet tails can be a normal finding. Typically these are limited to the last lateral intercostals space above the diaphragm with a hot spot often seen on the right most caudal anterior axillary window [22, 9]. Care must be taken, however, in attributing a hot spot in the lower lateral windows to a benign finding, as local lung consolidation from diseases such as ARDS, atelectasis, or pneumonia can exhibit this pattern. [22, 11]. In those cases, the clinical presentation of dyspnea with other physical signs and symptoms such as low oxygen saturations and fever should be used to help differentiate "normal" from diseased state. With the case of patients presenting with dyspnea, the pathologic state should be considered present until "ruled out" with other diagnostic modalities. However in the research arena where "healthy" subjects may be tested, the pre-test probability that comet tails localized to the last lateral intercostals spaces are normal, is high.

A diffuse bilateral comet tail pattern is not considered normal and is indicative of alveolar-interstitial syndromes (AIS). These can be brought about by a number of disease entities including chronic conditions such as pulmonary fibrosis, and acute entities such as acute respiratory distress syndrome (ARDS), interstitial pneumonia, and acute pulmonary edema [5]. Different clinical presentations can help elucidate the etiology of these different diseases which have the same comet tail pattern. The time course of the illness can differentiate chronic causes such as pulmonary fibrosis and acute causes such as pulmonary edema. Additionally slight variations in the pattern of comet tails are noted. In the case of a fibrotic lung, the comet tails are equal in both hemi thoraces, whereas in cardiac pulmonary edema they are bilateral but with a predilection for the right hemi-thorax. Also in the fibrotic lung comet tails are more patchy than in pulmonary edema, and are stable with diuretic therapy [9].

Highly dense entities such as ARDS typically give rise to comet tails only in regions where the diseased lung is in contact with the sub-pleural space. These highly dense areas give rise to multiple comet tails less than 3 mm apart, whereas comet tails arising from thickened inter-lobular septa are 7 mm apart [23]. Additionally an ARDS pattern also gives rise to comet tails in focal areas which coalesce together and form comet tails of differing lengths and multiple irregular comet tails [7, 23, 1].

Importantly comet tails which arise from pulmonary edema should respond to treatment and disappear as interventions are made [18]. If they do not, then an alternate diagnosis should be sought. This reenforces the need for serial exams many authors encourage repeat exams to monitor response to therapy.

Since the presence of the occasional comet tail is considered normal, the lack of comet tails can be diagnostic as well. Comet tail formation requires an area of differing acoustic impedances, when this is not present no comet tails are created. Such is the case of a pneumothorax. In examining for this potential emergent condition, an additional ultrasonographic sign must be viewed, that of the "sliding lung sign." This is the hyperechoic line which is the interface between the visceral and parietal pleura. This line will slide back and forth with respiration. When there is no sliding of this line, and an absence of comet tails, a pneumothorax should be suspected [24]. The is particularly helpful when some studies show that standard chest x-ray, in addition to taking longer, misses 30% of cases [25-27]. This is contrasted to the lung ultrasound which in a large meta-analysis and systematic review looked at 8 studies representing 1,048 patients. When using both the absence of lung comet tails and sliding lung sign ultrasound was 90.9% sensitive and 98.2% specific in making the diagnosis of pneumothorax. In the same analysis chest radiograph was only 50.2% sensitive, but with a similar specificity of 99.4% [28].

In patients with minimal comet tails confined to the intercostal space above the diaphragm, or no comet tails present on lung ultrasound, but who otherwise present with dyspnea, other common diagnoses should be considered. These include COPD, acute bronchitis, and pulmonary embolism [1]. The issue of COPD is a special consideration which has been studied by at least three groups. In the initial comet tail paper, Lichtenstein observed that COPD could give rise to a fibrotic pattern, bilateral comet tails [7]. However later work performed by the same author comparing ultrasound to x-ray diagnosis suggested that the presence of diffuse bilateral comet tails was absent in 92% of patient with COPD (N=26) and absent or confined only to the laster intercostal space in 98.75% of patients without respiratory disorder (N=80). The two patients in the COPD group who had a positive test (the false positives) had pneumonia in the regions viewed as positive on ultrasound. In the patients without respiratory symptoms, one patient demonstrated a positive test. Interestingly even though he did not have any symptoms, that one patient was admitted for acute renal failure requiring urgent dialysis, again supporting the idea that ultrasound findings occur before symptoms [22]. Additional studies also support the lack of findings of comet tails in COPD exacerbations. In fact in one study looking at the presence of comet tails in patients with acute shortness of breath, the most common discharge diagnosis of patients who did not exhibit bilateral diffuse comet tails was COPD [1, 18, 21].

Overall this technique allows for the rapid assessment of patients in respiratory distress and can take less than three minutes [9, 15]. When used for detecting pulmonary edema, it has nearly a 95% concordance with chest radiographs [1] and, as discussed above, may be more sensitive than chest radiograph for this diagnosis [15]. A gross recognition of the comet tail pattern present, as well as the patient's history and response to treatment can guide the clinician to the correct diagnosis. In terms of application, bedside ultrasound in many emergency departments and intensive care units is readily available.

6. Special situations

Due to its ease of use, portability and relative low cost, this technology is ideally suited for remote research and clinical applications. In fact a bedside ultrasound is the only diagnostic imaging currently used on the International Space Station.

Research applications have used the ultrasonographic finding of comet tails to monitor pulmonary edema in healthy volunteers subjected to extreme environments. These include ironman athletes, breath-hold deep divers, and mountain climbers [29]. Due to the remote nature of the conditions, ultrasound is especially useful in mountaineering where up to 10% of climbers above 4,000 M develop the life-threatening condition known as High Altitude Pulmonary Edema [30]. (See Figure 5) At an altitude of 4,240 M Fagenholz, using the CTS technique described in this chapter, showed that a CTS score of 35 +/- 11 corresponded to patients suffering from HAPE which differed from those who were short of breath from other causes who had a CTS of 12 +/-6.8 [20]. Others have shown that in the presence of normal left ventricular function and normal pulmonary artery pressures, sojourners above 4790 m can develop pulmonary edema with a corresponding decrease in oxygen saturation. The comet tails describe in these studies had right lung predominance [31]. When used in the high altitude environment, care should be taken to ensure that the device employed uses solid state storage.

http://dx.doi.org/10.5772/56198

This is found on most modern portable ultrasounds. Non-solid state devices cool using fans which will over heat at extreme altitudes.

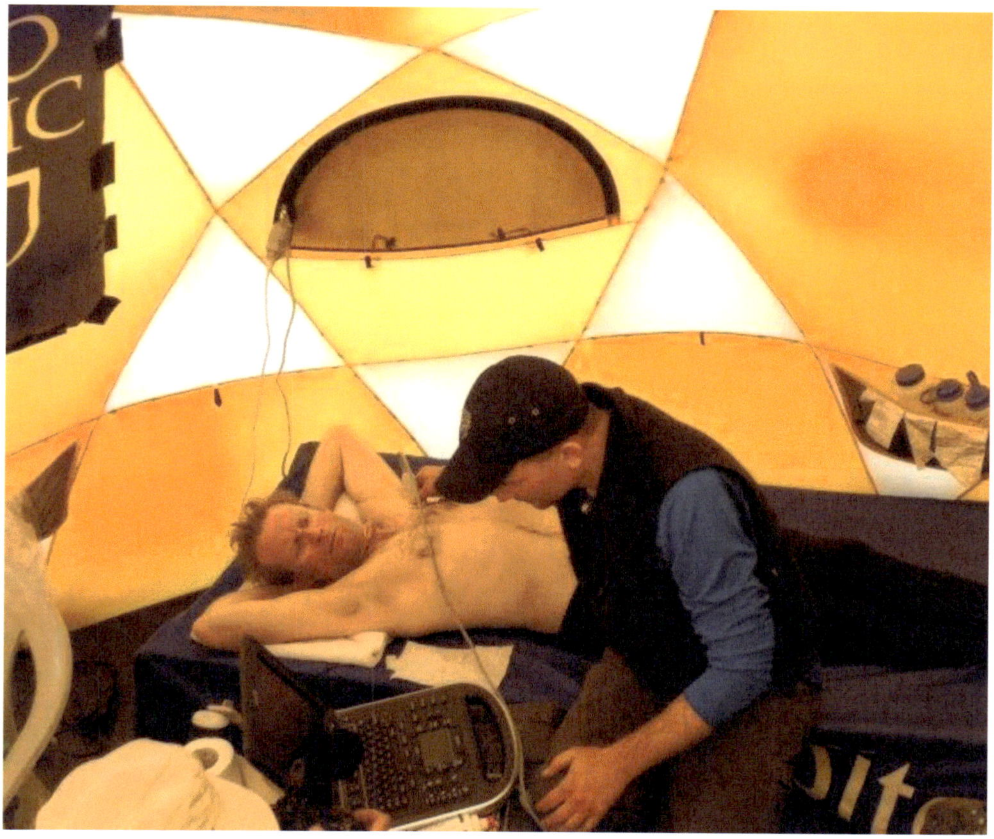

Figure 5. Author (DS) demonstrating the ease of use and portability of modern ultrasound systems by performing an assessment of EVLW at the base camp of Mt Everest, ele 5,364 M, on an elite climber.

7. Conclusion

Although dyspnea is a leading cause of hospital admission, determining its etiology and subsequent treatment remains one of the greatest diagnostic challenges a clinicians faces. While many have lamented the perceived loss of physical exam skills amongst practitioners, the traditional lung exam and classic findings heard on auscultation are often difficult to hear in a noisy intensive care unit or emergency department [32, 33]. Even in ideal circumstances, there is abundant literature to suggest that the physical exam may be inaccurate [14, 15]. This leads the clinician to rely on adjuncts to aid in diagnosis.

In the case of dyspnea, chest radiograph are typically employed to help narrow the differential diagnosis. However even these can be fraught with difficulties including time to obtain, and read the x-ray. Fortunately the field of ultrasound and echocardiography has greatly expanded in the past 20 years. The lung ultrasound finding of comet tails can help guide therapeutic interventions, and unlike chest radiograph, the exam can be repeated without fear of increased radiation exposure.

With the advent of small bedside machines, lung ultrasound techniques can become an extension of the physical exam. These exams can be repeated as often as necessary in response to changing clinical conditions. In this way ultrasonographers can guide real-time decision making for patient care.

Acknowledgements

Funded by grants from NIH HL71478, Mayo Clinic and The North Face Company.

Author details

Douglas T. Summerfield and Bruce D. Johnson*

*Address all correspondence to: Johnson.bruce@mayo.edu

Divisions of Pulmonary and Critical Care Medicine and Cardiovascular Diseases, Mayo Clinic Rochester, USA

References

[1] Zanobetti, Maurizia, et alCan chest ultrasonography replace standard chest radiography for evaluation of acute dyspnea in the ED?" Chest. (2011). , 139, 1140-1147.

[2] Wang, C. S, et al. Does this dyspneic patient in the emergency department have congestive heart failure?" JAMA. (2005). , 294, 1944-1956.

[3] Cremona, G, et al. Pulmonary extravascular fluid accumulation in recreational climbers: a prospective study." Lancet (2002). , 359, 303-309.

[4] Milne, E. N. et. al. "The radiologic distinction of cardiogenic and noncardiogenic edema." AJR Am J Roentgenol. (1985). , 144, 879-894.

[5] Volpicelli, Giovanni, et alBedside lung ultrasound in the assessment of alveolar-interstitial syndrome." American Journal of Emergency Medicine. (2006). , 24, 689-696.

[6] Levitov, A. Critical Care Ultrasonography. (2009). New York, New York: McGraw-Hill

[7] Lichtenstein, Daniel et alThe Comet-tail Artifact." Am J Respir Crit Care Med. (1997)., 156, 1640-1646.

[8] Ziskin, M. C, et al. The comet tail artifact." J Ultrasound Med. (1982)., 1, 1-7.

[9] Picano, E, et al. Ultrasound lung comets: A clinically useful sign of extravascular lung water." J Am Soc Echocardiography. (2006)., 19(3), 356-363.

[10] Kerley, P. Radiology in heart disease. BMJ (1933).

[11] Agricola, Eustachio, et alUltrasound Comet-tail images: A Marker of pulmonary edema: a comparative study with wedge pressure and extravascular lung water." Chest. (2005)., 127, 1690-1695.

[12] Lichtenstein, D. A, et al. A-lines and B-lines: lung ultrasound as a bedside tool for predicting pulmonary artery occlusion pressure in the critically ill." Chest. (2009)., 136(4), 1014-1020.

[13] Jambrik, Z, et al. Usefulness of ultrasound lung comets as a nonradiologic sign of extravascular lung water." Am J Cardiology. (2004).

[14] Tsverava, M, & Tsverava, D. Comet tail artefact in diagnosis of pulmonary congestion in patients with diastolic heart failure." Georgian Medical News. (2010)., 10(187), 28-35.

[15] Vitturi, N, et al. Thoracic ultrasonography: A new method for the work-up of patients with dyspnea." Journal of Ultrasound. (2011)., 14, 147-151.

[16] Stapczynski, J. S, et al. Congestive heart failure and pulmonary edema." Emergency medicine: a comprehensive study guide. New York: McGraw-Hill; (1992)., 216-219.

[17] Lange, N. R, & Schuster, D. P. The measurement of lung water." Crit Care. (1999). RR24., 19.

[18] Mallamaci, F, et al. Detection of pulmonary congestion by chest ultrasound in dialysis patients." JACC:Cardiovascular Imagin. (2010)., 3(6), 586-594.

[19] Staub, N. C. Pulmonary edema." Physiol Rev. (1974)., 54, 678-811.

[20] Fagenholz, P. J, et al. Chest ultrasonography for the diagnosis and monitoring of high altitude pulmonary edema." Chest., 131(4), 1013-1018.

[21] Volpicelli, G, et al. Usefulness of lung ultrasound in the bedside distinction between pulmonary edema and exacerbation of COPD." Emerg Radiol. (2008)., 15(3), 145-151.

[22] Lichtenstein, D, & Mezière, G. A lung ultrasound sign allowing bedside distinction between pulmonary edema and COPD: the comet-tail artifact." Intesive Care Med. (1998)., 24(12), 1331-1334.

[23] Lichtenstein, D, et al. Comparative diagnostic performances of auscultation, chest radiography, and lung ultrasonography in acute respiratory distress syndrome." Anesthesiology. (2004). , 100, 9-15.

[24] Lichtenstein, D, & Menu, Y. A bedside ultrasound sign ruling out pneumothorax in the critically ill. Lung Sliding." Chest. (1995). , 108(5), 1345-1348.

[25] Tocino, I. M, et al. Distribution of pneumothorax in the supine and semirecumbent critically ill adult." AJR Am J Roentgenol. (1985). , 144(5), 901-905.

[26] Chiles, C, & Ravin, C. E. Radiographic recognition of pneumothorax in the intensive care unit." Crit Care Med. (1986). , 14(8), 677-680.

[27] Ball, C. G, et al. Factors related to the failure of radiographic recognition of occult posttraumatic pneumothoraces." Am J Surg. (2005). , 189(5), 541-546.

[28] Alrajhi, K. Test characteristics of ultrasonography for the detection of pneumothorax: A systematic review and meta-analysis." Chest. (2012). , 141(3), 703-708.

[29] Garbella, E, et al. Pulmonary edema in healthy subjects in extreme conditions." Pulm Med. (2011).

[30] Bärtsch, P, et al. Respiratory symptoms, radiographic and physiologic correlations at high altitude." In: Sutton JR, Coates G, Remmers JE, editors. Hypoxia: the adaptations. Toronto: B.C. Decker;(1990). , 241-245.

[31] Pratali, L, et al. Frequent subclinical high-altitude pulmonary edema detected by chest sonography as ultrasound lung comets in recreational climbers." Crit Care Med. (2010). , 38(9), 1818-1823.

[32] Mccullough, P. A. Uncovering heart failure in patients with a history of pulmonary disease: rationale for the early use of B-type natriuretic peptide in the emergency department." Acad Emerg Med. (2003). , 10, 198-204.

[33] Remes, J. Validity of clinical diagnosis of heart failure in primary health care." Eur Heart J. (1991). , 12, 315-321.

Chapter 4

Ischemic Mitral Regurgitation: From Echo Assessment to Surgical Strategy and Techniques

Gheorghe Cerin, Adrian Bogdan Popa,
Razvan Ticulescu and Marco Diena

Additional information is available at the end of the chapter

http://dx.doi.org/10.5772/56062

1. Introduction

Ischemic mitral regurgitation remains an underestimated and important clinical problem. It is a complex multifactorial disease that involves global and regional left ventricular remodeling as well as dysfunction and distortion of the components of the mitral valve including the chordae, annulus and leaflets. The prevalence rate of development of mild or more severe degree of mitral insufficiency after myocardial infarction has been estimated to be up to 50% and is associated with worse prognosis (Stevenson 1987, Lamas 1997, Grigioni 2001).

Based on the clinical presentation, the ischemic mitral regurgitation was classified as acute or chronic (Mitesh, 2009). Although the acute ischemic mitral regurgitation is relatively rare, whenever present, it has a rapid evolution, with an extremely poor survival rate. On the other hand, the chronic ischemic mitral regurgitation is much more frequent, but it's the consequence of a slower pathological process, with a better survival rate. The echocardiography identifies all patterns of ischemic mitral regurgitation; nonetheless the classification as acute, sub-acute or chronic ischemic mitral regurgitation is rather clinical, than an echocardiographic one. Beside the complete rupture of papillary muscle, other patterns of ischemic mitral regurgitation cannot be practically located in time by echo. It is possible to have the same echocardiographic feature of the lesion in acute and in chronic settings; only the clinical presentation of the patient helps in the diagnosis of acute / sub-acute or chronic ischemic mitral regurgitation. So the echo exam has to be seen as complementary to clinical data, rather than a singular method of diagnosis.

In everyday practice the management of ischemic mitral regurgitation represents a combined problem of physiopathology, quantification and diagnosis that, together, drive the individual patient prognosis but, in case of patients candidate to open heart surgery this becomes a very complex issue. With intraoperative TEE echocardiography, the exact identification of the mechanism of ischemic mitral regurgitation represents a cornerstone element for surgical planning and patient management. In case of significant residual mitral regurgitation a second run of the extracorporeal circulation may be necessary requiring a well-founded experience from the echocardiographer as the TEE intraoperative findings may be sometimes misleading.

The relation between the ischemic mitral regurgitation, surgery and echocardiography, as tool for surgical planning and postoperative control, will be addressed in this chapter. The suboptimal results obtained by the most commonly used surgical strategy, that is, restrictive annuloplasty combined with coronary artery bypass graft, emphasizes the need to develop alternative or concomitant surgical techniques that directly target the causal mechanisms of the disease. Recent data show that this procedure is associated with a 10% to 20% rate of persistent mitral regurgitation soon after operation and a 50% to 70% rate of recurrent mitral insufficiency at five years (Hashim 2012, Magne 2009). Hereafter, the topics will be focused mainly on the echo assessment of the patients candidate for open-heart surgery. A particular attention will be paid to the papillary muscle and to the mitral valve geometry and their role in the pathophysiology of ischemic mitral insufficiency. Understanding the mechanisms of the different types of ischemic mitral regurgitation is mandatory for echocardiographer and surgeon to tailor the right strategy for the valve repair, and it is indeed a challenging task for both.

2. Physiopathology: Concepts regarding post-myocardial left ventricular remodeling, acute and chronic ischemic mitral valve and the valve geometry

It is generally assumed that the ischemic mitral regurgitation is not a valve disease, the *'engine'* of valve insufficiency being the remodeling process of the left ventricle, depending on the localization and extension of the myocardial infarction. In ischemic heart disease, the mitral leaflets (and also the chordae) are typically structurally normal, but the leaflets are tethered and their motion is relatively restricted, owing to regional and global ventricular remodeling, with apical displacement of the posteromedial papillary muscle.

Sometimes the remodeling process starts immediately after the onset of myocardial infarction causing structural ischemic mitral regurgitation, which is associated with a poor prognosis, due to the concomitant acute infarction, acute papillary muscle remodeling and **acute ischemic mitral regurgitation**. For a successful management of this acute mechanical complication the key point is the early diagnosis, which has to be done before the complete rupture of the papillary muscle occurs. This life-threatening complication has otherwise to be considered a failure due to late echocardiographic and clinic diagnosis.

Overall, there is only scanty literature concerning the echocardiographic assessment of the papillary muscle and it is no surprising then to see that its use in the everyday practice is, so

http://dx.doi.org/10.5772/56062

far, very limited. There are only few general recommendations and the guidelines do not include them in the systematic evaluation of the ischemic mitral regurgitation. Most of the current information focuses on regional and global ventricular remodeling, with leaflets tethering and tenting, motion restriction and annular dilatation. Frequently, the ischemic remodeling of papillary muscle is difficult to document; nevertheless with an accurate analysis, often performed in non-standard echocardiographic views, the diseased papillary muscle may be identified.

In coronary patients with mitral insufficiency, beside the ventricular remodeling, annular dilatation and leaflets (mobility and tethering), the echocardiographer has to focus the attention on the shape, the length and the thickness of the papillary muscle, mainly in acute circumstances, when the acute remodeling process is just beginning (fig 1).

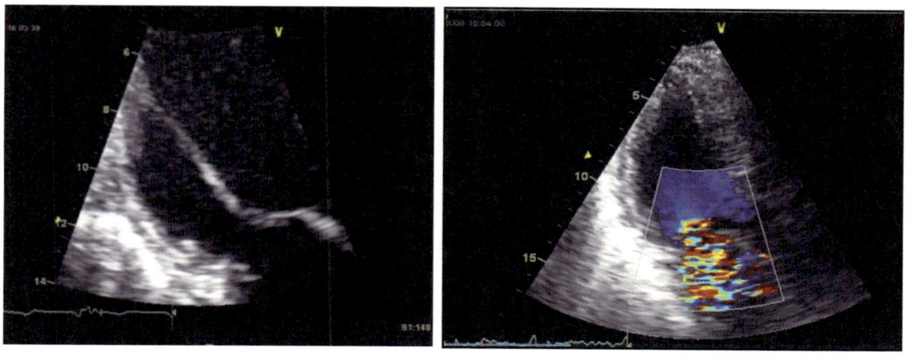

Figure 1. Acute inferior MI with severe MR due to acute post-ischemic elongation of PP MM. Note the abnormal length and shape of the very slim PP MM. The tip reaches the level of the MV annular plane. Often (as in this case), the elongation PP MM is visible in a different plane respect of the MR at color Doppler. MI = myocardial infarction; MR = Mitral regurgitation; PP MM = papillary muscle; MV = mitral valve.

On the other hand, in the case of **chronic ischemic mitral insufficiency**, all the remodeling processes of left ventricle causing the ischemic mitral regurgitation are slower, the evolve over time and usually the echo diagnosis is not so tricky. Generally, the patterns of chronic ischemic mitral regurgitation are quite often the same: tethering of the papillary muscle, chordae and leaflets, various degree and progressive dilation of the left ventricular cavity and mitral annulus, mitral valve tenting, with reduced / loss of coaptation and restriction of one or both leaflets (fig 2, 3). The post-infarction loss of the contractile ventricular mass is directly correlated with the remodeling process, expressed by the heart dilatation and decreasing of cardiac reserve. All the elements belonging to the mitral apparatus will be involved in this process, but the leaflets and the chordae are, as a matter of fact, preserved.

Ischemic mitral regurgitation has several pathophysiological determinants. It has been defined as a ventricular disease that affects the mitral apparatus, because both myocardial infarction and ischemia generate progressive global and regional left ventricular remodeling, and consequently, a functional mitral regurgitation. Apical and posterior displacement of the papillary muscle is a typical echocardiographic finding. This process starts ordinarily with the

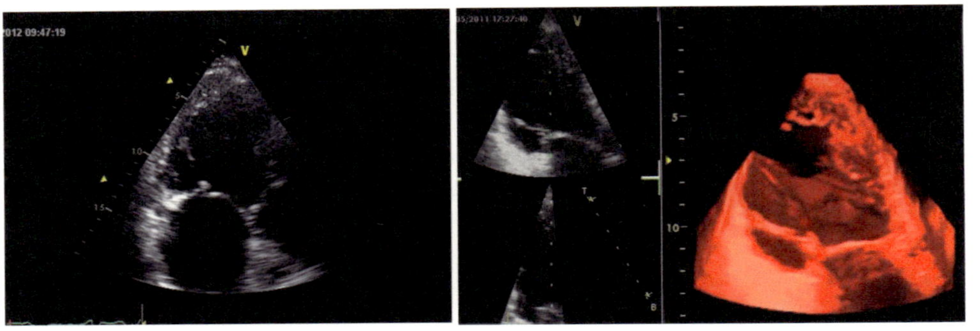

Figure 2. Inferior myocardial infarction with ischemic mitral regurgitation due to systolic restriction of posterior mitral leaflet (2D and 3D systolic frame, from two different patients). Note the systolic tension on the chordae belonging to the posterior mitral valve with limited excursion of the cusp, the asymmetrical apposition of the anterior leaflet and the reduced area of coaptation.

posterior leaflet because the posterior mitral annulus is thinner, weaker, more flexible and without a zone of resistance. On the contrary, the anterior leaflet has a more thickened and less malleable annulus. In this way the posterior leaflet became firstly restricted while the anterior is involved only later on. The echocardiography is able to assess the relationship between the LV cavity (shape, dimensions, volume), the mitral leaflets (as mobility, leaflet apposition, length and height of coaptation, annulus dimension, etc) and the valve geometry.

In the case of chronic ischemic mitral regurgitation and ischemic dilated cardiomyopathy, (generally patients with anterior and inferior infarction), the right balance between the dimension of the mitral valve and the 'new' dimension of the double infarcted ventricular cavity is lost, so that the mitral valve becomes insufficient. Conceptually, it may be assumed that there is a phenomenon of *'mismatch'* between the *'too large'* left ventricle and *'too small'* mitral valve apparatus, which is unable to extend the drapery of the leaflets and to adapt to the new dimension of the infarcted ventricle (fig 3). That's why, in case of critical coronary artery disease leading to left heart dilatation and ischemic mitral regurgitation, the 'standard' surgical approach of coronary artery by-pass grafting (CABG) plus undersized ring alone, may not solve completely the mitral regurgitation and, over time, the repair may fail (Magne 2009). In these cases the annuloplasty ring alone is not enough to achieve sufficient *'fabrics'* for a stable coaptation and repair. Ideally speaking, to get a good repair more tissue is needed to enlarge the mitral valve. This concept will be addressed in the chapter of chronic ischemic mitral regurgitation.

The chronic ischemic mitral regurgitation is classified as a *III°b type* of mitral insufficiency essentially due to the systolic restriction of the posterior leaflet (Table 1). The practice demonstrates that in the case of ischemic mitral regurgitation this classification may be incomplete and misleading because the chronic ischemic mitral regurgitation has always a combined annular dilation of the valve, which in fact is a type I° mechanism of mitral regurgitation in Carpenter's classification (Carpentier 1983 & 2010). That's why, for a better and more precise diagnosis of the mechanisms of ischemic mitral regurgitation, **the mitral valve geometry** has to be carefully assessed.

http://dx.doi.org/10.5772/56062

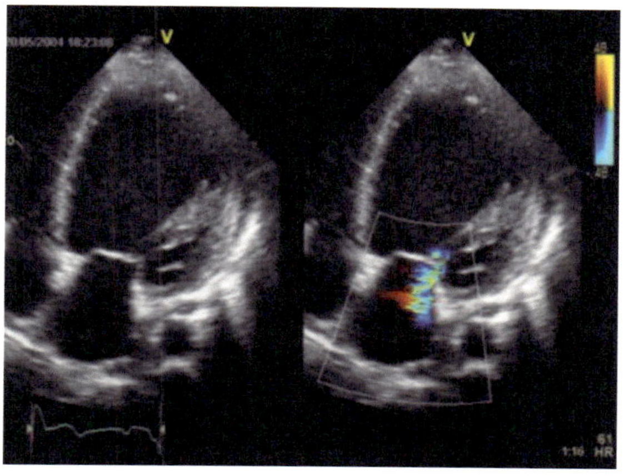

Figure 3. Ischemic dilated cardiomyopathy and the concept of "mitral - ventricular mismatch" (see the text). Patient with double myocardial infarction (anterior and inferior).Ischemic dilated cardiomyopathy and chronic ischemic mitral insufficiency. Note the spherical shape and dilatation of the left ventricular cavity, the reduced surface of coaptation of mitral leaflet (2mm), due to the annular dilatation (41mm) and the laterally migration of the papillary muscle.

Type I°	Normal leaflet motion
Type II°	Excess leaflet motion (leaflet prolapse)
Type III°	Restricted motion
$III°_a$	Restricted opening
$III°_b$	Restricted closure

Table 1. Carpentier's classifications of Mitral Regurgitation

As noted (Cerin 2006, Tesler 2009), from the geometrical point of view, the normal mitral valve presents *a triangle* delimited between the coaptation point (typically sited inside of the ventricular cavity) and two others referral points, placed on the anterior and posterior mitral annulus (standard pattern of a normal mitral valve – Fig 4). This *echocardiographic virtual tool* demonstrates to be useful in judging the mitral valve structural and functional abnormalities (Cerin 2012). When the echocardiographic presentation of ischemic mitral regurgitation is consistent with obvious deformation of this virtual triangle, this should raise the suspicion of a possible papillary muscle abnormality with elongation of sub-valvular apparatus, alongside to reduce / loss of leaflet coaptation.

In some cases the geometry of the mitral valve may be so distorted that an elongation of the sub valvular apparatus has to be suspected or is clearly present. In these particular cases, the echocardiography examination has to be focused on the papillary muscle lesions; this might require the execution of the exam in several off axis views, beside the standard ones. Patients with distortion of mitral valve geometry (fig 5A) will not fit within the III°b of Carpentier's classification. Some of these patient may present a clear ischemic mitral valve prolapse (type II° Carpentier), but many of them will show only a distortion of the 'standard' mitral valve triangle, with the coaptation point still present inside of the left ventricular cavity. The

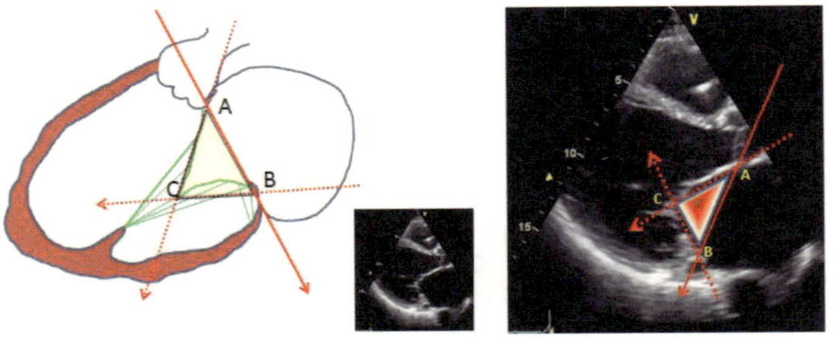

Figure 4. The coaptation triangle and the mitral valve geometry. The normal pattern of mitral valve anatomy and function is characterized by the triangle of coaptation which is defined by the coaptation point (C), normally sited inside of the left ventricular cavity and two other points (A, B) placed on the anterior and posterior mitral annulus.

geometrical analysis of these patients will show the disappearance of the mitral valve triangle and a progressive the transformation of it in a *'trapeze'*. (Fig 5B).

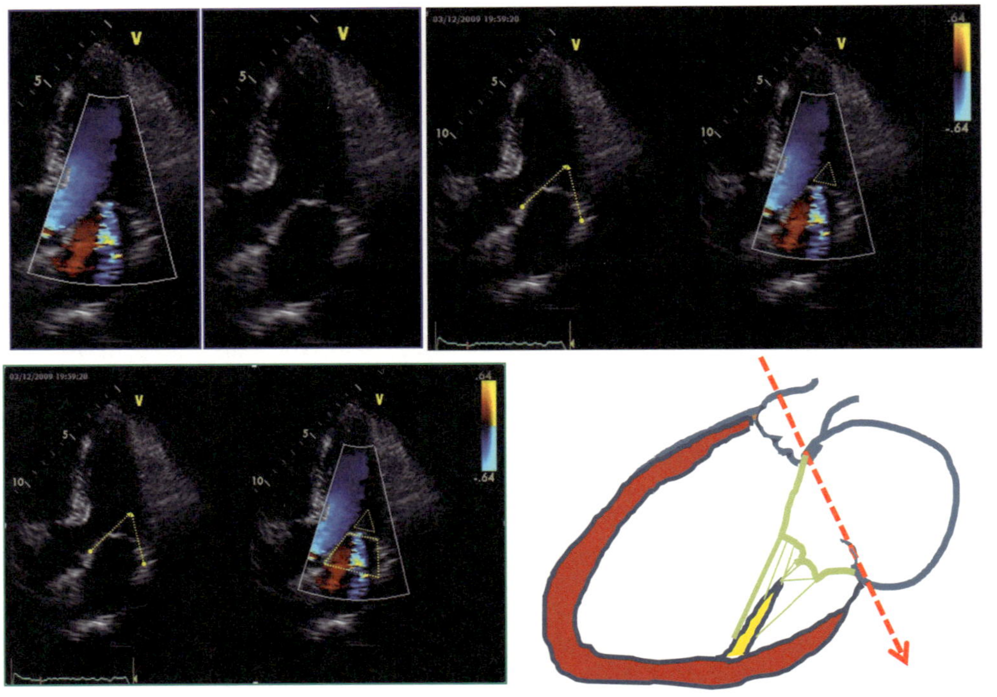

Figure 5. A (up) and B (down). Ischemic mitral regurgitation with **distorted mitral valve geometry**. Note the absence of the 'standard triangle of coaptation' which as a matter of fact was transformed into a 'trapeze' due to the post-ischemic 'crash' of the edge of the mitral valve, generated by papillary muscle elongation (drawing).

The repair strategy by the undersized rings alone may not solve the mitral regurgitation in patients with distorted mitral valve geometry (due to papillary muscle elongation). This because the small ring corrects the mitral annulus deformation only, whereas the main problems of these patients are represented by the displacement of coaptation plane too 'high', nearby the mitral annulus, the distortion of the coaptation surface and plane due to the 'crash' of the tip of the mitral valve tenting and the reduced mitral leaflet coaptation (fig 5B, scheme). The mechanism of regurgitation in these patients is clearly more complex than the classical 'leaflet restriction' (III°b type of Carpentier's classification).

Often the mechanisms involved in the ischemic mitral regurgitation are multiple, complex and intricate, and the surgical planning of the valve repair must to be tailored, ignoring partially and sometimes totally the classifications; classifications often focus on the mitral leaflet only (which are practically normal) and do not include the papillary muscles, the mitral valve geometry and the grade of general or regional left ventricular remodeling.

Depending of the clinical context, a check list of the echocardiographic elements has to include: dimension of the left ventricular cavity (as diameter and volume), diameter of the mitral annulus (transthoracic, PSLAx systole), the sphericity index and the distance between the papillary muscle (in case of ischemic cardiomyopathy), the length of leaflets coaptation, the length of the anterior leaflet, the 'height' of the posterior leaflet, the mobility of the anterior and most of all the posterior leaflet, etc.

From this point of view, beside of the others elements involved in valve regurgitation, the use of the *triangle of coaptation* as tool of mitral valve geometry (Cerin 2010) shows to be a suitable instrument 'to judge' better the mechanisms of ischemic mitral regurgitation (Fig 4, 5A, 5B). In some cases, due to obviously papillary muscle elongation, the triangle may completely disappear (see the Fig 6).

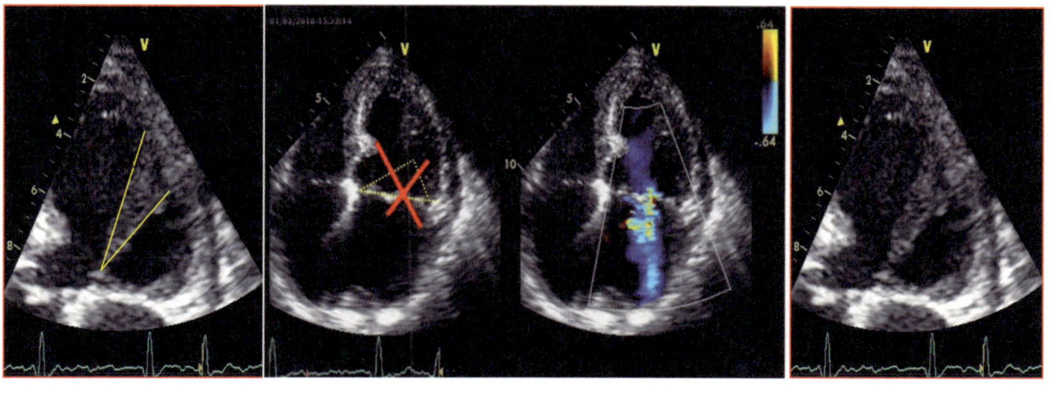

Figure 6. Chronic ischemic mitral regurgitation, due to reduce leaflet coaptation (approx. 2mm), dilatation of the left ventricle (EDVol 245ml) and of the mitral annulus (Ø45mm). Note the absence of 'the coaptation triangle' due to ischemic elongation of papillary muscle: the length of papillary muscle is completely unusual, having the tip situated very near to the mitral annulus. Note also the triangular shape of this muscle, with a very sharp tip, due to progressive post-ischemic remodeling with elongation: so called 'thorn papillary muscle'. Because of the abnormal post-ischemic elongation of the papillary muscle, the normal geometry of mitral valve was distorted and the triangle of coaptation disappears. NB – all the images belong to the same patient.

The echocardiographic assessment of the mechanisms of the ischemic mitral regurgitation, which is the key for the tailored surgical approach, may be sometimes complex and tricky, due to a true mosaic of intricate mechanisms, difficult to be embedded and defined by a standard classification. The echocardiographer has to be aware of the complexity of the left ventricular remodeling process and to assess the mitral valve apparatus using multiple views and to pay particular attention to the analysis of the mitral valve geometry.

3. Acute ischemic mitral regurgitation

Background. Acute ischemic mitral valve regurgitation may occur in the setting of acute myocardial infarction owing to necrosis and rupture of papillary muscle tissue or abnormal coaptation of the leaflets, due to distortion of ventricular geometry. Hemodynamically significant mitral regurgitation is possible in both anterior and inferior infarcts, but its incidence appears higher in the inferior myocardial infarction group such as 40% vs 15% - see the Fig 7 (Estes 1966, Dagum 2000, Timek 2003). Post-infarction mitral regurgitation may be associated to multiple cardiovascular risk factors such as diabetes, abnormal body mass index (>25), advanced age, female gender, coexistence of peripheral arteriopathy and prior infarction (Green, 1999).

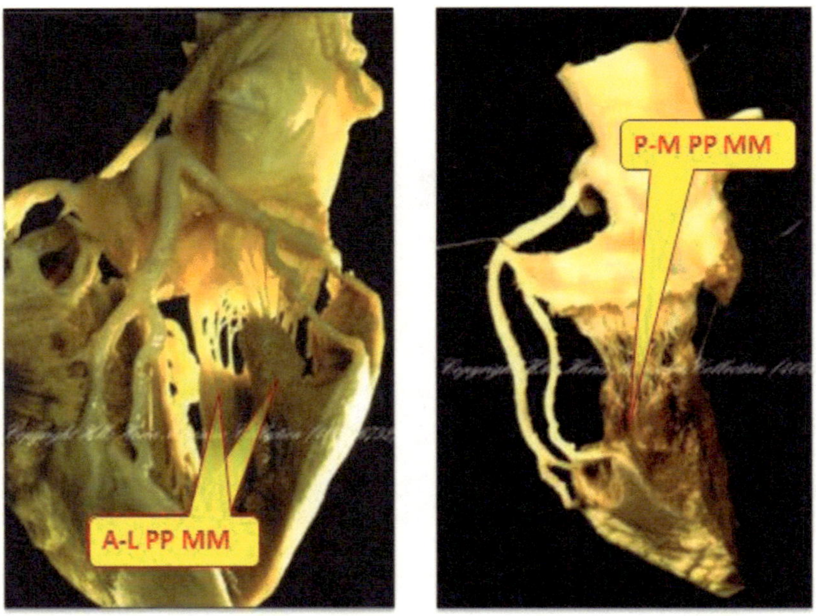

Figure 7. Differences in the vascularization of the papillary muscle. Postero-medial papillary muscle usually receives the blood only form the right coronary artery (rarely from circumflex artery), respect of the antero-lateral papillary muscle which has two sources of vascularization: left anterior descending artery and circumflex artery. By courtesy of MURESIAN Horia, MD, PhD - 2009.

http://dx.doi.org/10.5772/56062

The acute ischemic mitral regurgitation (Fig 8) is more often due to structural lesions as complete or partial rupture of the papillary muscle, and less frequent due to an elongation of the muscle. The echocardiographic diagnosis may not be easy and it is often based on the use of the TEE in the emergency facility. The key issue in the successful management of these patients is timely intervention. If the clinical conditions and the logistic allow it, the patient should be urgently taken to the operating room. Most often, the acute ischemic regurgitation is surgically treated by mitral valve replacement. Mitral valve repair is rare, but, in specific cases, it may be a valid alternative. This depends on the quality and on the entity of the structural alteration of the subvalvular apparatus, and also on the experience of the surgical team.

From the echocardiographic point of view, the acute structural ischemic mitral regurgitation may present three different patterns: transection of papillary muscle ("too late" diagnosis), partial rupture of the papillary muscle ("timely" diagnosis) and elongation of the papillary muscle (the "tricky" echo diagnosis); see the scheme on the Fig 8.

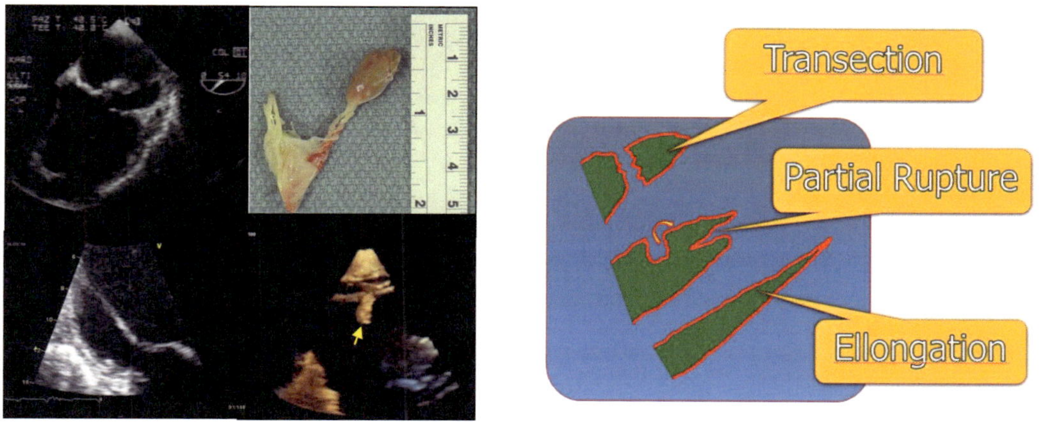

Figure 8. Echocardiographic classification of the structural acute ischemic mitral regurgitation (scheme). The upper pictures represent a case with transection of papillary muscle, in a patient with cardiogenic shock ("too late" echo diagnosis). In the bottom raw acute papillary muscle elongation (the first pictures on the left) and partial rupture of papillary muscle (right picture, yellow arrow); both patients were in 3rd NYHA Class.

The gloomy clinical prognosis of acute significant ischemic mitral regurgitation associated to myocardial infarction (moderate or severe degree) is illustrated by its devastating impact on short- and long-term survival: almost one out of 4 patients die at one month and more than one out of 2 after one year (24% early and 54% 1-year mortality rate) (Otto, 2012).

In most cases the acute ischemic mitral regurgitation is a syndrome with conspicuous clinical implications. Generally, the clinical presentation of these patients is compatible with a hyper acute heart failure; they are highly symptomatic and may present with overt acute pulmonary edema, cardiogenic shock or even sudden death. Only minorities of patients are mildly symptomatic or asymptomatic and may present just a new systolic murmur.

Based on the echocardiography exam the acute ischemic mitral regurgitation may be divided in structural and functional. The structural ischemic mitral regurgitation is determined by complete papillary muscle rupture (transection), by partial detachment of one or both tips of a papillary muscle with subsequent elongation and by acute remodeling of papillary muscle with elongation (fig 8). In some cases the ischemic event may involve the point of insertion of the tendineous chord(s) which may result in a 'flail' which is an uncommon pattern for this pathology but may explain this kind of lesion.

In summary a myocardial infarction, in acute settings, may have one of the three structural damages on the papillary muscle: transection, partially rupture or elongation. The first two situations have already largely been described in many publications. This is not the case with the papillary muscle elongation, which is closer to chronic ischemic regurgitation and where the echocardiographic geometrical analysis, based on *the triangle of coaptation,* plays an essential role in diagnosis.

3.1. Papillary muscle necrosis with complete rupture of papillary muscle

Papillary muscle necrosis with complete rupture of papillary muscle is an uncommon but dramatic type of ischemic mitral insufficiency, with approx. 1.0% incidence in patients with myocardial infarction (Clements 1985). This is a life-threatening complication of myocardial infarction that requires a prompt diagnosis and surgical intervention (Fig 9). The posteromedial papillary muscle is more frequently involved because of its single coronary artery blood supply (Fig 7). Chordae to both leaflets arise from each papillary muscle so that, in cases of "complete" rupture, both leaflets are affected. The echocardiography exam generally shows loss of leaflets coaptation due to the floating ruptured papillary muscle ('flail' mitral valve). In these patients the echocardiographic diagnosis is relatively simple and, generally, may be done using transthoracic exam. These patients belong to the type II° Carpentier's classification.

Nonetheless the complete rupture is rare; it carries a poor prognosis for the onset of acute pulmonary oedema and low output syndrome. Without surgery, the mortality is very high, up to 75% within the first 24 hours (Tcheng, 1992, Kirklin 2012). As a consequence, the echocardiographic diagnosis must rapidly be performed and the patient must be timely taken to the operating room. In most cases the intervention is a mitral valve replacement. However the operative mortality is high, ranging from 23 to 45%, increasing in late referral. It may reach 57% in cases of reoperations (Loisance, 1990).

3.2. Incomplete papillary muscle rupture

Sometimes the papillary muscle is only partially ruptured. To avoid the high operative mortality in case of complete papillary muscle rupture, the diagnosis of papillary muscle rupture has to be done on this circumstance. Usually the clinical manifestation of this condition is an episode of acute heart failure occasionally with a relative stabilization and sometimes with a new systolic murmur. The echocardiographic diagnosis may be available using the transthoracic approach, but might also be relatively tricky and then the TEE should be preferred for the reasons mentioned above (unstable patient, unclear transthoracic view).

The echocardiographic presentation of this type of structural ischemic mitral regurgitation generally shows a prolapse of one leaflet; also the type II° Carpentier's classification (which in

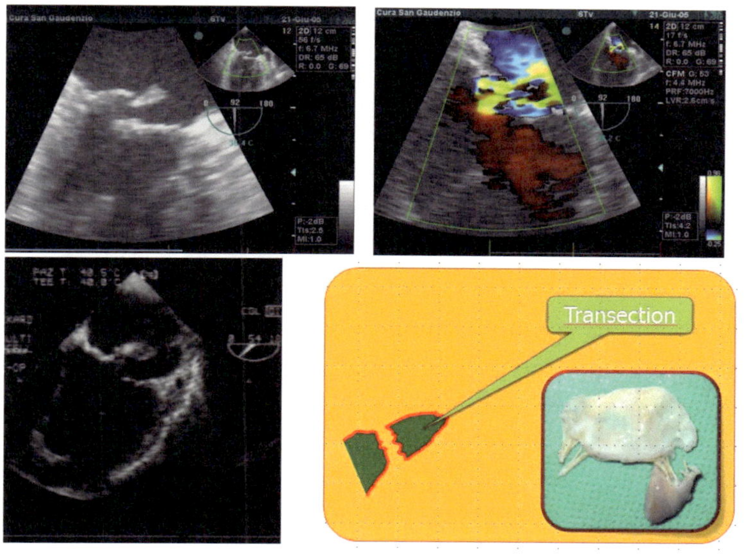

Figure 9. Acute severe structural ischemic mitral regurgitation due to transection of papillary muscle (2D TEE intraoperative exam). Note the loss of coaptation due to complete rupture of papillary muscle and flail (arrows). Both patients, with hemodynamic instability, were transferred to Cardiac Surgery Dpt. the same day of the transthoracic diagnosis. An emergency mitral valve replacement and CABG was successfully performed after coronary angiography.

reality is a *'false'* mitral valve prolapse). An asymmetric apposition of the *'prolapsed'* leaflet is also present. Often these patients are misdiagnosed as *'mitral prolapse'*, because the echocardiographer focuses the attention only on the mitral valve, neglecting to assess the papillary muscle. So, it is possible to fall into the trap, because at variance from the mitral valve, the papillary muscle is generally seen in a different echocardiographic plane, and often off axis view. If the echocardiographer doesn't have the concept of possible elongation of the papillary muscle due to the structural post-necrotic lesion, the true etiology of the lesion may be missed (Fig 10).

The take home message is to check explicitly the papillary muscle, searching it from different off axis views, starting from the clinical settings of the patient, essentially in case of abnormal geometry of the mitral valve. At any transthoracic suspicion of partial papillary muscle rupture the TEE exam must be done, chiefly in acute settings. The partial papillary muscle lesion may be otherwise missed and it may evolve to a complete rupture. At the echo, the ruptured head shows a hypermobile, redundant excursion which may mimic a degenerative lesion (e.g. Barlow disease). It is critical to remember that in most cases of papillary muscle involvement, massive mitral regurgitation is present and the surgery must be rapidly accomplished (Fig 11). In some cases mitral valve repair is possible depending on the intraoperative findings, the elapsed time from the acute myocardial infarction and the surgeon experience.

3.3. Acute remodeling of the papillary muscle with elongation

Acute remodeling of the papillary muscle with elongation is the third and rare form of acute ischemic mitral regurgitation which, usually, involves the inferior-posterior papillary muscle.

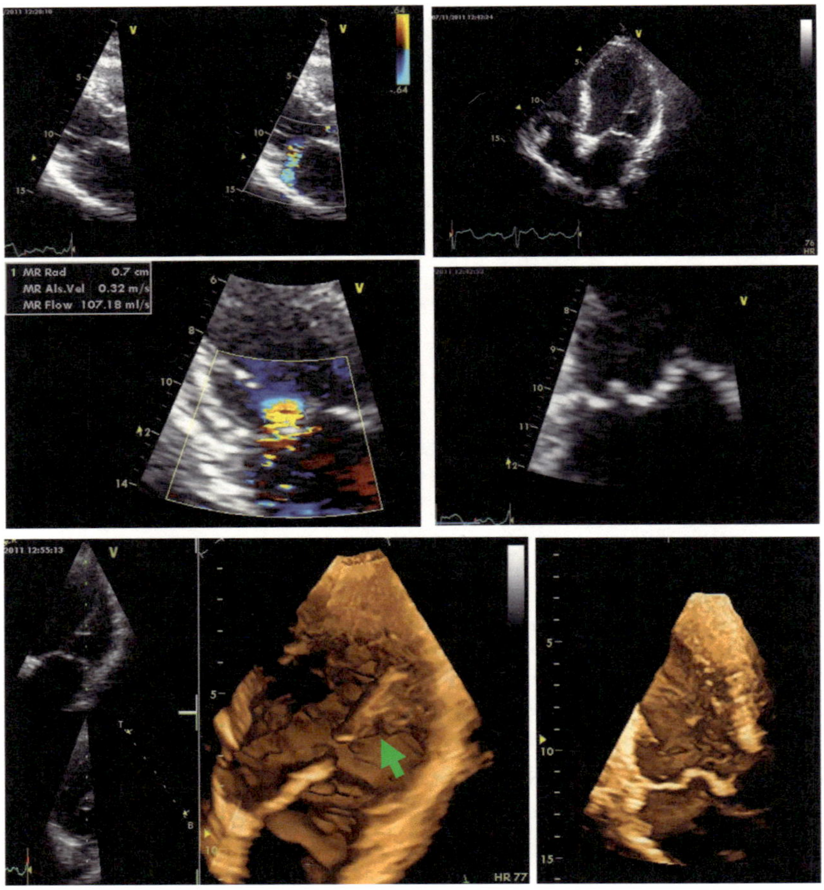

Figure 10. Ischemic mitral regurgitation due to acute elongation of papillary muscle, appearing as mitral valve prolapse. The pictures on the middle raw show prolapse of both mitral leaflet. In reality, only the focused examination on the papillary muscle shows the triangular shape of the muscle, with a sharp tip and a partial tearing beside (arrow, bottom raw, 3D TTE).

At the echo, the papillary muscle has a triangular shape and appears elongated and often slim (fig 12). This elongation determines a displacement of the coaptation point towards the mitral annular plane and to the left atrium, with subsequent mitral regurgitation. In this way the appearance of mitral valve is likewise similar with the mitral valve prolapse (type II° Carpentier classification), but the etiology is the myocardial necrosis and not the anomaly of the connective tissue as in Barlow / Marfan disease.

The echocardiographic documentation of the ischemic etiology in these cases might be tricky. In order to better characterize the structural anatomy of the myocardium at the level of the infarcted or ischemic papillary muscle, additive methods could prove useful such as SPECT, cardiac MRI or PET, showing the myocardial scar or necrosis. Anyway, the diagnosis is extensively based on the geometrical analysis of the mitral valve apparatus performed by echocardiography.

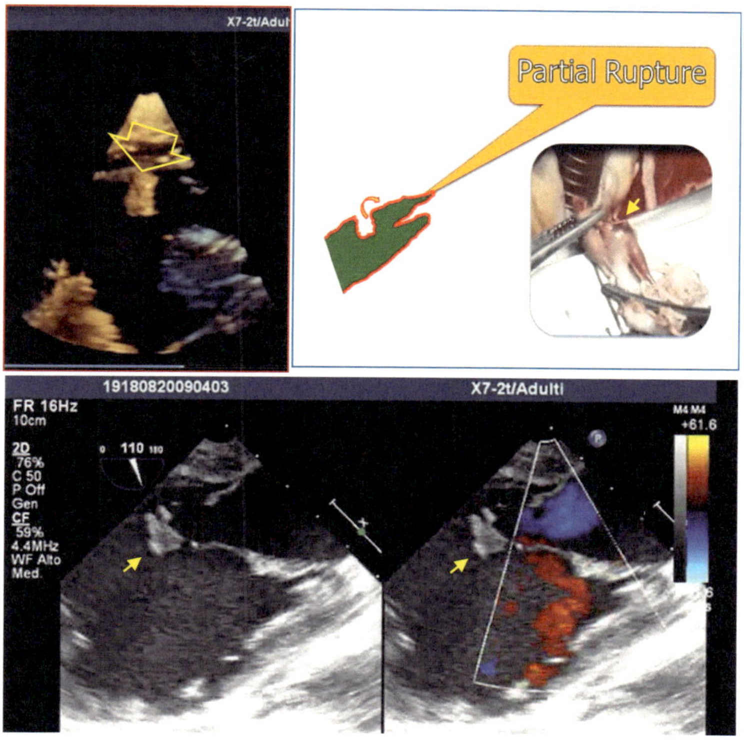

Figure 11. Partial rupture of papillary muscle (yellow arrows); TEE 3 D and 2 D exam and intraoperative picture.

The echocardiographic presentation of these patients shows a mitral valve with excess leaflets motion and prolapse, having the coaptation point situated *'very high'* near the mitral annulus, due to an elongated papillary muscle. If the papillary muscle is difficult to visualize, the virtual tool of *triangle of coaptation* may be useful to suppose the true etiology, considering that the normal geometry of the mitral valve will be distorted, with disappearance of the standard triangle.

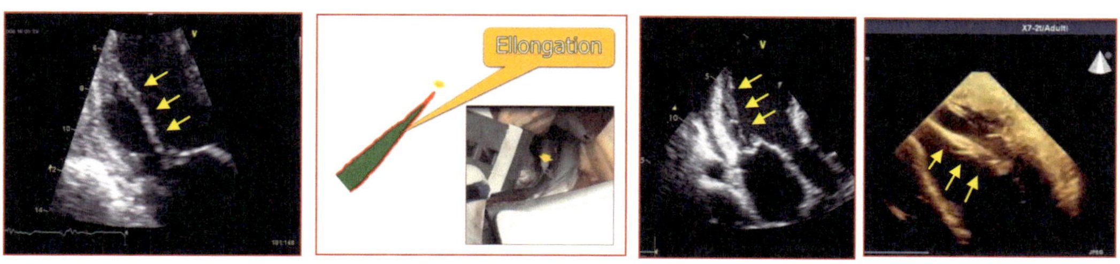

Figure 12. Acute post-ischemic elongation of papillary muscle (yellow arrows); scheme, intraoperative photo and 2D and 3 D Echo. Note the tip of the papillary muscle (in the intraoperative picture and Echo slides) which reaches at the level of the mitral annulus. The papillary muscle is very thin, with a slim triangular shape and a very sharp tip: 'thorn papillary muscle'. In all cases the mitral valve presents severe regurgitation. Note the absence of the triangle of coaptation, due to the migration of the coaptation plane nearby the mitral valve annulus.

The proper diagnosis and thus the management of such a serious clinical condition as the acute ischemic mitral regurgitation must rely on clear and robust echocardiographic concepts such as mitral valve geometry and functional anatomy. As already said the normal mitral valve geometry is the standard that guides both the evaluation of the various valve lesions and the surgical treatment. The central feature of the normal mitral valve geometry is represented by **the triangle of coaptation** (fig 4). The coaptation length (CL) and the coaptation height (CH) are cornerstone elements used in order to fully describe the valve geometry and to assess the result of the repair (Cerin 2012). It may be assumed that from a three dimensional geometrical perspective the triangle of coaptation corresponds roughly to an asymmetrical tent. In the course of perioperative echocardiographic study, the systematical analysis of the mitral valve apparatus is done, focusing on whether the triangle of coaptation is present or not. This geometrical concept of the mitral valve allows the repair to be performed even in some of the serious cases of acute mitral regurgitation.

Nevertheless, it should be underlined that this condition, even if rare, is a very severe cardiological emergency, often characterized by low cardiac output and high early mortality; with medical therapy about 90% of patients with acute ischemic mitral regurgitation will died in the first two months. This is the reason why surgical correction must not be delayed. The predictors of better survival are: early operation, short duration of shock and mild degree of left/right ventricular impairment. For the management of these patients the use of intra-aortic balloon pumping and / or ventricular assist device (fig 13), out of inotropic pharmacologic support, is mandatory. Surgery might be delayed up to 2-3 weeks only when patient is stable; in this setting, as noted, the surgery is performed with lower risk.

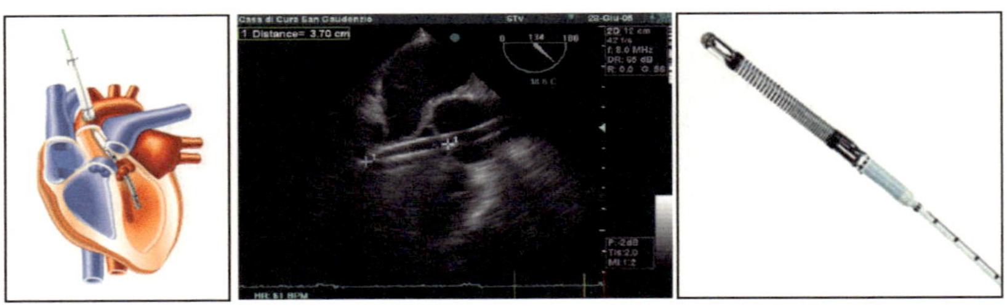

Figure 13. Acute heart failure due to ischemic mitral regurgitation. TEE intraoperative picture showing the assessment of the right position of the ventricular assist device (Impella) into the left ventricular outflow tract.

4. Chronic ischemic mitral regurgitation

4.1. Physiopathological consideration

Largely, the chronic ischemic mitral regurgitation is considered a long-lasting developing process of LV remodeling after myocardial infarction, causing mitral regurgitation by dysfunction and distortion of the components of the mitral valve including the chordae, the annulus and the leaflets. Nevertheless, this is not always true: some patient with acute

http://dx.doi.org/10.5772/56062

infarction may develop an *acute* and dynamic process of ventricular remodeling involving the papillary muscle, which may not be perceived or checked in real time at echo and discovered later, as *'chronic'* mitral regurgitation.

From this point of view, the classification of ischemic mitral regurgitation in acute and chronic may be in some cases misleading; ischemic mitral regurgitation is a ventricular disease, following the same steps as the myocardial infarction. So, as the myocardial infarction recognizes an acute period, a recent (sub-acute) and then a stable (chronic) phase, it seems logical to use the same classification for ischemic mitral regurgitation. In the era of shorter hospitalization of infarcted patients the acute ischemic mitral regurgitation, being a dynamic phenomenon, may be missed at the first echo examinations and 'discovered' over time, as 'late' complication (Popa BA 2007) (fig 14); Thus, the echocardiographer has to be aware that the classification in acute or chronic may reflect mainly the moment of diagnosis and less the true period of time when the lesion occurred. This aspect is important as regard the prognosis of ischemic mitral regurgitation, because, as noted, the acute and sub-acute ischemic mitral regurgitation have a worse prognosis over a short period of time, respect of chronic ischemic mitral regurgitation.

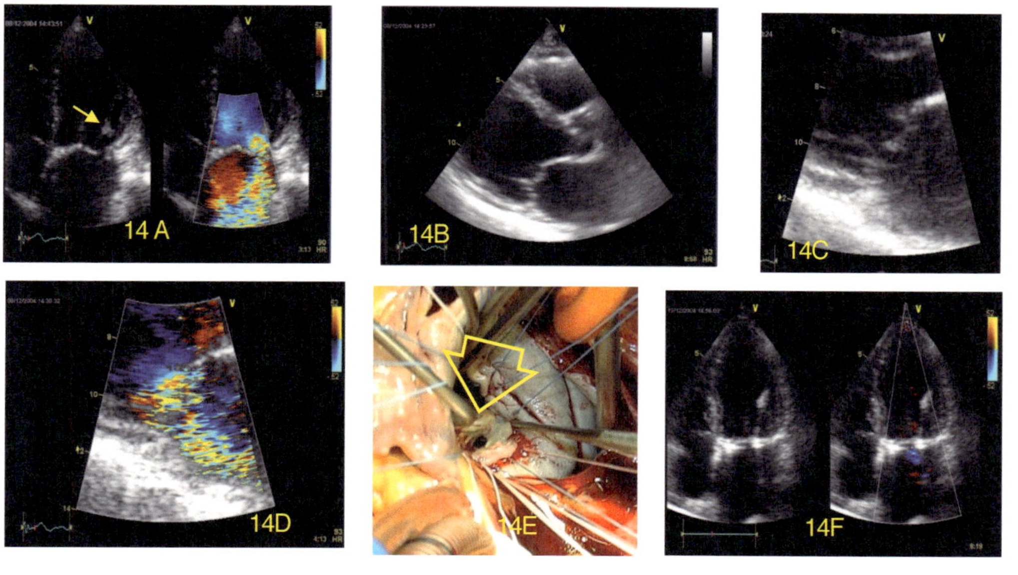

Figure 14. Severe ischemic mitral regurgitation (14D) diagnosed by TTE 10 years after an acute 'uncomplicated' myocardial infarction. The clinical presentation of the patient was exertion dyspnea. Ten years before, at discharge from the hospital the Echo exam has been normal. Note the elongation of the papillary muscle (14 A,C,E), causing loss of leaflet coaptation (14 A,C), with marginal prolapse of A_2 scallop (14B,C). Apparently the patient presents an A_2 localized prolapse (14BC), which, in reality is caused by an elongated papillary muscle. The tip of the papillary muscle is shown (14E, yellow arrows), arriving till the mitral annular plane (which is categorically abnormal). The transthoracic postoperative echo after mitral repair (mitral ring + suture and shortening of the papillary muscle), shows trivial residual mitral regurgitation (14F).

The chronic ischemic mitral regurgitation, comparing with the acute one, is a much more gradual and more complex process, because of the slow progression over time of the left heart remodeling (fig 14). This clinical condition recognizes two main mechanisms: a structural alteration of the subvalvular apparatus (papillary muscle and the corresponding LV wall), alongside of the phenomenon of left ventricular cavity remodeling.

4.2. Left ventricle post infarction remodeling process

From the physiopathological point of view the left ventricular post myocardial infarction remodeling is considered to be a phenomenon which can be divided in two parts: a regional and a global process of remodeling.

Regional remodeling is more often found after the inferior infarction (but not only), and may evolve over time in two different ways:

1. mainly a process of inferior wall remodeling with displacement of the papillary muscles. This type is associated with overt systolic restriction of posterior mitral leaflet.
2. inferior wall remodeling and displacement of the papillary muscles, *combined with post-ischemic elongation of papillary muscles*. In this kind of inferior post infarction remodeling the systolic restriction of the posterior mitral leaflet may be less evident or even absent in some cases. Respect of the first type, the geometry of mitral valve in this sort of ventricular remodeling will be different.

Global left ventricular remodeling is generally seen after two heart attacks (multiple myocardial infarctions and in cases with ischemic dilated cardiomyopathy) and it is characterized by restriction of both mitral leaflets, tethering of the mitral valve apparatus with mitral valve tenting, due to progressive migration of the papillary muscles simultaneously with overall left cavity dilatation.

In the patients with left ventricular remodeling and chronic ischemic mitral regurgitation, these physiopathological concepts are expressed by **two main echocardiographic patterns of left heart remodeling:**

a. the echocardiographic pattern of **limited LV remodeling:** inferior or lateral infarction scar, mild left ventricular dilatation, mild systolic dysfunction and chronic ischemic mitral regurgitation due to unambiguous systolic restriction of posterior leaflet (fig 15), and
b. the echocardiographic pattern of **extensive LV remodeling:** major left ventricular cavity dilatation with dysfunction and distortion (by anterior and inferior myocardial infarction), typically with poor systolic function, but also with a diastolic one and the tethering of both mitral leaflets (fig 3).

Both types of chronic ischemic mitral regurgitation present a mitral annular dilatation, obviously more evident in patients with double myocardial infarction. A form of *symmetric remodeling of the mitral valve apparatus* is present in patients with ischemic dilated cardiomyopathies ('extensive' LV remodeling) due to bilateral migration of *both* the papillary muscle (scallops P_1/P_2/P_3). Conversely, a limitary process of mitral valve apparatus remodeling is present in patients

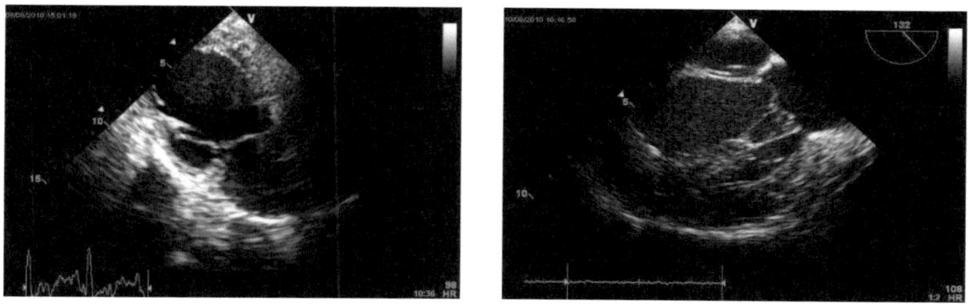

Figure 15. Limited LV remodeling: TTE (left) and TEE 2-chamber view (right) showing systolic restriction of the posterior mitral leaflet and minimal leaflet coaptation. Necrosis of the inferior wall is evident, with mild left ventricular dilatation (EDVol 170ml), mild systolic dysfunction (EF 43%) and chronic ischemic mitral regurgitation due to clear systolic restriction of posterior leaflet.

with 'limited' LV remodeling (inferior infarction) and *asymmetric mitral valve remodeling*, due to *solitary* migration of the postero-medial papillary muscle (scallops P_3/P_2).

These two main echocardiographic patterns of LV remodeling, when associated with chronic ischemic mitral regurgitation, are easy to identify by transthoracic echocardiographic exam and the transesophageal examination is not necessary. Sometimes, these configurations may be less definite, as in patients with regional or global remodeling, combined with coincident papillary muscle elongation. In these cases there is an additional phenomenon of migration of the LV infarcted wall, associated with post ischemic elongation of the papillary muscle.

A geometrical analysis of the mitral apparatus, by use of the echocardiographic tool of *triangle of coaptation* may identify these patients with regional or global remodeling, combined with elongation of the papillary muscle. As already has been mentioned, the patients with papillary muscle elongation present a distortion of the triangle of coaptation with progressive alteration of the standard trilateral shape (fig 5), till the complete disappearance of it (fig.6). The mechanism of mitral insufficiency in these patients is more complex and the surgical strategy has to be tailored accordingly.

The elongation of the papillary muscle may often be unnoticed if the operator mostly focuses the attention on the mitral leaflet, on the valve coaptation and on the degree of mitral regurgitation. Moreover, the papillary muscles are difficult and rarely seen in the same plane with the mitral valve leaflets, being sited distant from the coaptation valve plane; only a specific and vigilant off axis assessment of them may reveal the muscularly post-ischemic remodeling.

When the papillary muscles elongation is obvious, the surgical strategy has to be adapted and sometimes a shortening of them or use of the artificial chordae may be necessary to restore a good plane of valve coaptation and valve geometry.

Therefore, as message for the everyday practice, in acute or in chronic ischemic mitral regurgitation, the marker of the papillary muscle elongation is the distorted coaptation triangle.

Consequently, in the analysis of ischemic mitral regurgitation the starting points are restricted motion of the posterior mitral leaflet (type III° Carpentier's classification), combined with mitral annular dilatation, secondary to migration of the wall and left ventricular enlargement (fig 15). The consequent mitral regurgitation leads to left ventricular volume overload, closing the vicious circle of ischemic mitral regurgitation and of left ventricular remodeling. The echocardiographic examination will show the tethering of one or both mitral leaflets, which is the 'standard' pattern of chronic ischemic mitral regurgitation. However, around 10% of patients with chronic ischemic mitral regurgitation may show a different pattern of regurgitation with 'false mitral prolapse', by elongation of the papillary muscle due to local ischemia, necrosis and/or fibrosis (false because the etiology is not degenerative, but ischemic one).

In these patients, from the echocardiographic point of view, there are three elements that may suggest the suspicion of ischemic etiology of the prolapsed valve:

1. leaflets - prolapse limited to one of the mitral leaflets, often of the anterior one,
2. papillary muscle - specific appearance of the papillary muscle: elongated, hyperechogenic, thinning and triangularly shaped; *"thorny"* papillary muscle (fig 16);
3. valve geometry - the abnormal mitral valve geometry, with distortion of the triangle of coaptation, until its complete extinction (see also the Fig 5, 6)

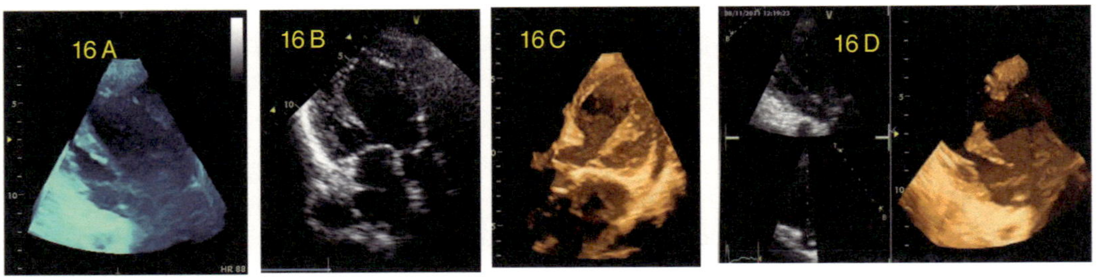

Figure 16. A,B,C,D. Four different cases with chronic post ischemic elongation of the papillary muscle: 2D transthoracic exam (16B) and live 3D (A,C,D). Note the progressive thinning of the papillary muscle, with the sharp aspect of the tip of it: so called 'thorny papillary muscle'.

Chronic ischemic mitral regurgitation may also be synonymous with ruptured tendineous chordae. Due to ischemia or necrosis the insertion place of the mitral chords on the tip of the papillary muscle may become friable, and often a limited *'ischemic flail'*, may be apparent (fig 17).

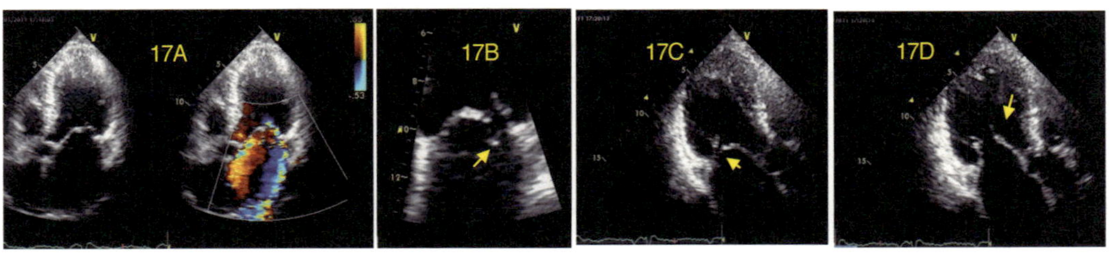

Figure 17. Loss of leaflet coaptation (B,C), with flail (B) and eccentric jet. The free ruptured chordae is visible in systole (C) and also in diastole (D). The pictures belong to the same patient.

http://dx.doi.org/10.5772/56062

Indication to surgery: With an ever increasing population of patients with coronary artery disease complicated by chronic ischemic mitral regurgitation, the question whether to perform a mitral valve repair in addition to CABG is one of the most common and controversial clinical dilemmas faced by cardiac surgeons and cardiologists today. There is a general agreement regarding the indication for surgery in patients with severe ischemic mitral regurgitation. The problem arises for moderate ischemic mitral regurgitation. At present, there is no definitive randomized, prospective trial that clarifies which approach should be taken. The 2011 ACCF/ AHA guidelines on CABG state that patients undergoing CABG who have severe ischemic mitral valve regurgitation not likely to resolve with revascularization, should have concomitant mitral valve repair or replacement at the time of CABG (Class I, Level of evidence B) (Gillinov 2001, Trichon BH 2003, Fattouch K 2009 & 2010, Zoghbi W 2003). Operative mortality is considered to be around 10% (Rankin 1988, Cohn 1995, Grossi 2001). Some studies advocate mitral valve repair to all patients that undergo CABG even when the degree of mitral regurgitation is mild. This strategy seems to be reasonable if the chronic ischemic mitral regurgitation is considered to be expression of the LV deformation / remodeling process, which is not still reversible in the chronic phase of the myocardial infarction. A careful echocardiographic analysis focused mainly on the quality of leaflet coaptation and on the extension of LV deformation (limited or extensive remodeling), may guide the surgeon.

5. Assessment of ischemic mitral regurgitation severity

Due to the hemodynamic conditions in ischemic heart disease and the particular shape of the regurgitant orifice, assessment of the severity of mitral regurgitation may be challenging. Mitral regurgitation in an ischemic setting has a profound impact on patient's prognosis and therefore its quantification plays a key role in the revascularization plan because moderate and severe mitral regurgitation have indication to surgery. Given this special impact on prognosis, the thresholds of defining a severe mitral regurgitation in ischemic patients are much lower than in other contexts (see below the PISA method).

The qualitative method, based on regurgitant jet area, is not reliable. This is true especially when an exact assessment of mitral regurgitation is need, because this approach is prone to many biases, being so dependent upon loading conditions and on equipment settings (for example color gain). The gradient between left ventricle and left atrium will highly influence the size of the jet. In an acute mitral regurgitation, in which left atrium pressure is elevated and the left ventricle-left atrium gradient is low, the regurgitant jet may be small, even though the real regurgitant volume is important. Conversely, in a high blood pressure setting (i.e. a high left ventricle-left atrium gradient) the regurgitant jet will be bigger. Last but not the least, eccentric jets (like the ones found in posterior leaflet restriction), seem smaller than the central ones due to Coandă effect (hugging of the adjacent wall of the left atrium).

The semi-quantitative (vena contracta) and **quantitative methods** (PISA) are therefore advisable whenever their determination is possible.

Vena contracta is the narrowest region of the regurgitant jet, which is found not at the level of the leaflets, but just below the regurgitant orifice (because the blood is still converging for a few millimeters before re-expanding in left atrium) (fig 18). Its width is a marker of the regurgitant orifice area. It should be measured in a window perpendicular to the coaptation line, like parasternal long axis or four chambers views. A value of < 3mm is compatible with a mild regurgitation, while a value of >7mm is indicative of severe regurgitation. Values in-between are not diagnostic of a moderate mitral regurgitation, because of an important overlap. In ischemic mitral regurgitation, the shape of the regurgitant orifice is not round, but rather elliptic. For this reason, assessment of vena contracta width should be done in two orthogonal planes (e.g. parasternal and apical four chambers) and an average of these two should be reported. A value > 8 mm is diagnostic of severe regurgitation. The 3D echo can be a solution for assessment of vena contracta in an ischemic setting.

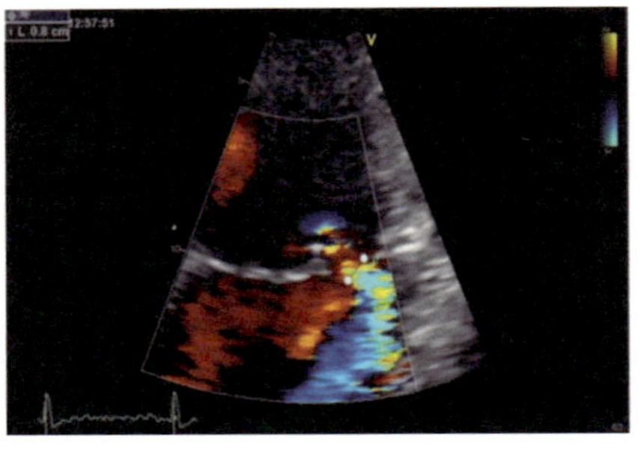

Figure 18. Vena contracta depth measurement at the narrowest point of the regurgitant jet. The three components of the jet are visible: convergence zone, vena contracta and the flow into the left atrium.

Quantitative approaches and especially PISA (proximal isovelocity surface area) are the most indicated. PISA is based on the fact that near the regurgitant orifice, the blood (which should pass throw a restricted area) is disposed in hemispheric layers, having the same velocity at a certain distance from the orifice. Lowering the Nyquist limit at 15-40 cm/s (the velocity at which aliasing is appearing), all the "layers" with a higher velocity will have the aliasing phenomenon. Measuring the first aliasing hemisphere we'll have a marker of regurgitation degree.

PISA method permits assessment of:

- **the flow rate** (FR) as $FR = 2 \times \pi \times R^2 \times Val$

where *R* is the PISA radius and *Val* is the aliasing velocity

- effective regurgitant orifice area (ROA) as *EROA=FR/V max*

where *FR* is the flow rate and *V max* is the maximum velocity measured on mitral regurgitation envelope in continuous Doppler

- **regurgitant volume** (RV) as *RV=ROA x TVI*, where *EROA* is effective regurgitant orifice area and *TVI* is the time-velocity integral measured on mitral regurgitation envelope in continuous Doppler (fig 19).

http://dx.doi.org/10.5772/56062

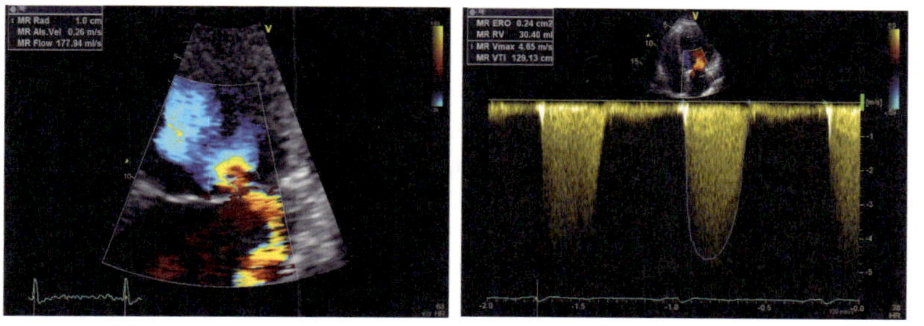

Figure 19. Assessment of mitral regurgitation severity according to PISA method (MR ERO, MR Flow). The baseline of color Doppler is moved toward the regurgitant jet direction and the hemisphere radius is measured (left). On the mitral regurgitation envelope (continuous Doppler) maximum velocity and TVI are determined

In eccentric jets (posterior leaflet restriction) the largest PISA is to be found in the parasternal long axis view, while in central jets the apical four chambers view should be used.

The elliptic shape of regurgitant orifice found in ischemic mitral regurgitation leads the PISA method to underestimate the real regurgitant volume (PISA is bigger than a hemisphere). Considering the profound deleterious effect of mitral regurgitation in an ischemic context, cut off levels of severity are lower than in organic mitral regurgitation, i.e. an EROA more than $20mm^2$ (vs. >$40mm^2$ in organic mitral regurgitation) and a regurgitant volume greater than 30ml (vs. >60ml) defines a severe ischemic mitral regurgitation.

Due to the dynamic characteristic of ischemic mitral regurgitation, PISA is not the same throughout the whole systole, being usually smaller in mesosystole when the regurgitation tends to decrease.

If hemispheric floor is not flat (i.e. 180º), an angle correction can be made. In this situation

EROA adjusted=EROA x $\alpha/180$, where α is the angle of convergence.

In multiple jets, both vena contracta width and PISA method are not additives and cannot be used.

Surgical approaches. Overview. The surgical treatment of acute or chronic ischemic mitral regurgitation is strongly influenced by the echocardiographic assessment, which remains the only tool for surgical planning and postoperative control. The complex mechanisms of ischemic mitral regurgitation are analyzed by echo and the surgical planning is done after transthoracic and usually elaborate after intraoperative transesophageal examination. Based on echocardiographic analysis, various approaches have been proposed for the management of ischemic mitral regurgitation. So far, both medical treatments and classical surgical techniques are not always sufficient. Within the next paragraphs a rapid overview of some of the various surgical techniques implied in the treatment of ischemic mitral regurgitation will be done.

1. **Undersized mitral valve annuloplasty.** The strategy of over-reduction of mitral annulus, combined with the coronary by-pass surgery is the most diffused surgical approach, especially in patients with dilated heart and chronic ischemic mitral regurgitation. As

noted, this technique addressed just the annular dilation. The echocardiographic examination plays an essential role because it confirms the dilation of the mitral annulus, and the subsequent reduced and/or loss of leaflet coaptation in case of advanced left ventricular and annular dilatation ('extended' LV remodeling pattern). As a rule, Echo indicates the presence of tethering of the mitral leaflets, and also the systolic and, in cases with advanced heart remodeling and ischemic dilative cardiomyopathy, the diastolic restriction of the posterior mitral leaflets.

Concomitant coronary revascularization and downsizing of the mitral annulus by prosthetic rings, showed promising results with 80% good competence of the mitral valve at 2-years follow-up, but only 50% at five years (McGee, 2004, Klein 2011). Better results were published by Dion (2004) according to a proper algorithm. Patients treated with this technique showed almost always the echocardiographic picture of the so-called "monoleaflet" mitral valve, where the anterior leaflet covers the entire mitral orifice and the posterior leaflet remains restricted in its diastolic position. At the time of surgery the preoperative TEE Echo assists the surgical mitral repair by estimating the length of the medial scallop of the anterior mitral leaflet (scallop A_2). This is usually performed from the distal-esophageal 135° view (three chamber view) and is essential in choosing the size of the annuloplasty ring. The choice of the size of the prosthetic ring is still empirical, but usually a ring two to three sizes smaller than measured is used.

The other determinant of the ischemic mitral regurgitation in the advanced stage of left ventricular remodeling is the restricted motion of the posterior mitral leaflet and loss of the anatomical and functional leaflet reserve both in systole and also in diastole. The existence of the anatomical and functional reserve of posterior mitral leaflet is a key element for having a competent mitral valve and, unfortunately, this aspect is not resolved by the over-reduction technique alone. To overcome the leaflet restriction some authors cut a limited number of basal chordae tendinae with the intent of reducing leaflet tethering and improving the coaptation. This simple procedure reduced tenting without creating valve prolapse, and the consequence is a decrease in mitral regurgitation (Messas 2001).

2. Because of these unsatisfactory results with the undersizing technique alone, the **repositioning of the posterior papillary muscle** has been proposed, mainly in patients with ischemic dilated cardiomyopathy, as adjunctive approach to the annuloplasty; the outcome is currently under evaluation (Hvass 2010). The role of intraoperative TEE is to define the deformation of the subvalvular apparatus from the geometrical point of view. On one hand, it must preoperatively assess the distance between the base of the papillary muscles (usually from the transgastric short axis view), and on the other hand it has to evaluate the geometry of the left ventricle using the sphericity index.
3. **Elongation of the posterior mitral leaflet with pericardial patch** (LEX), represents a relatively novel surgical approach to relief ischemic systolic restriction, despite some controversy regarding this technique (fig 20). Some encouraging results of LEX were reported but the number of treated patients is, so far, very limited (Dobre 2000, Langer 2006, de Varennes 2009). Surgical leaflet extension by autologous pericardial patch addresses directly the problem of ischemic leaflet restriction and tethering (type III°b

Carpentier classification). It is a physiologically coherent and relatively simple approach, intended to increase the surface and the mobility of the posterior mitral leaflet, in order to allow a better leaflet coaptation.

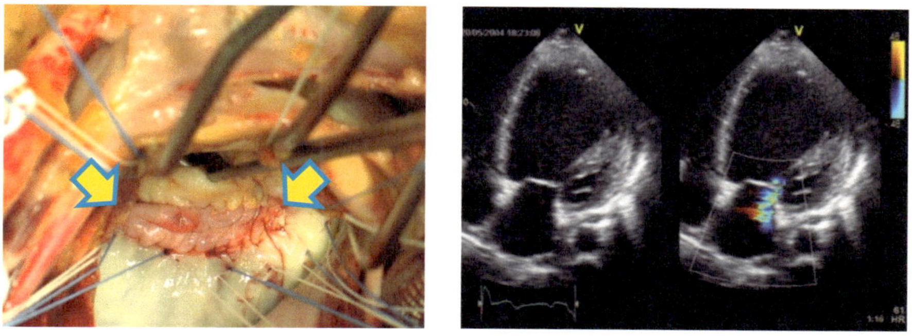

Figure 20. Posterior mitral leaflet after extension with pericardial patch (arrows) in a patient with ischemic dilated cardiomyopathy: extended LV remodeling (intraoperative view - left and TTE preoperative picture; right).

This technique allows the extension of the surface of the posterior leaflet, especially in the area of the scallops P_3 and P_2, which is normally more restricted by the post-ischemic tethering. Furthermore, this procedure provides an additional anatomical leaflet reserve: in case of continuing left ventricular remodeling after surgery, which may be present in about 50% of the patients, according to some authors. Leaflet extension by autologous pericardial patch has been widely and successfully used in the reconstruction of other mitral valve pathologies such as rheumatic disease and endocarditis, with acceptable long-term results (Zegdi, 2007). This procedure can be performed within 15-20 extra minutes of aortic cross-clamping, and allows implanting larger sizes mitral prosthetic rings, with minor diastolic gradient through the mitral valve. Further studies with larger number of patients and adequate long-term follow-up are needed to assess the efficiency of this simple and promising approach to the treatment of ischemic mitral regurgitation, in case of ischemic dilated cardiomyopathy.

Once more the echo plays an essential role by identifying the patient candidates to LEX. Typically the Echo aspect demonstrates small posterior mitral leaflets, systolic and, sometimes, diastolic leaflets restriction, with significant mitral regurgitation due to reduced coaptation and asymmetrical apposition of the anterior leaflet. Consequently, at the postoperative examination Echo evaluates not only the mitral valve function as expressed by the degree of residual regurgitation, but, more important, the anatomical (leaflet length) and functional reserve (the coaptation length).

For every day practice three main situations will be considered:

1. Chronic ischemic mitral regurgitation determined by restriction of the posterior leaflet and apical displacement of the papillary muscle in patients with inferior myocardial infarction (or inferior and lateral myocardial infarction), mild left ventricular dilatation and mild systolic dysfunction: so called 'limited' LV remodeling pattern.

2. Chronic ischemic mitral regurgitation by systolic (and sometimes diastolic) restriction of mitral leaflets motion (tethering of mitral leaflets) in patients with history of double or multiple infarction, overt left ventricular dilatation and depression of systolic function (ischemic cardiomyopathy): 'extended' LV remodeling pattern.

3. Chronic ischemic mitral regurgitation by papillary muscle elongation (with various degree of false prolapse of the mitral leaflets) (Hashim 2012); usually patients with inferior myocardial infarction, chronic ischemic mitral regurgitation and *distortion of the coaptation triangle.*

5.1. Chronic ischemic mitral regurgitation due to restriction

Chronic ischemic mitral regurgitation due to restriction of the posterior mitral leaflet and asymmetrical apposition of the anterior one, by apical displacement of the posterior papillary muscle and left ventricular wall. Fig 21.

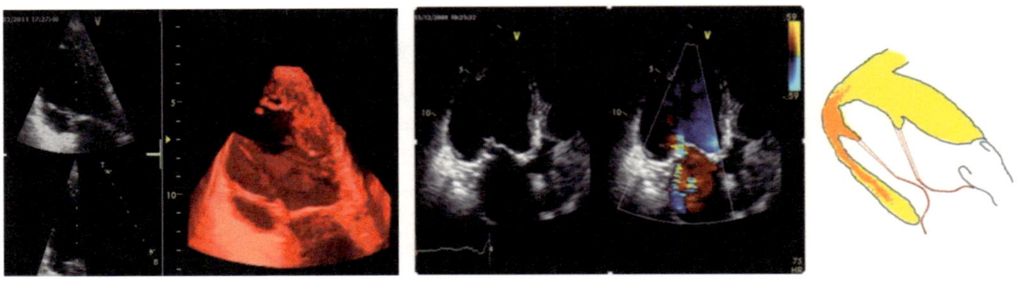

Figure 21. Systolic restriction of posterior papillary muscle; 3D and 2D transthoracic echocardiography and drawing.

Background. This is the most common type of ischemic mitral regurgitation (about 2/3 of all cases of chronic ischemic mitral regurgitation), belongs to the Carpantier's type III°b classification and has been extensively described. The valve leakage is here the result of alteration of subvalvular apparatus secondary to left ventricle remodeling following myocardial infarction. Frequently, they present with a myocardial scar caused by a previous myocardial infarction and the remodeling process of the left heart is less expressed, with mild systolic dysfunction. Respect of patients with ischemic dilated cardiomyopathy, this category of patients has less dilatation of the left ventricular cavity, and, as a rule, history of inferior (or lateral) myocardial infarction: echocardiographic pattern of limited LV remodeling. An infarction at the basal side of the left ventricle, involving the postero-medial papillary muscle will lead to a posterior and apical displacement of the papillary muscle, which will pull the posterior leaflet toward the posterior wall, impeding it to arrive to the normal coaptation plane during systole (figure 22). The postero-medial papillary muscle is more prone to ischemic remodeling than the antero-lateral one, having only a vascular source (from circumflex or right coronary), while the latter has a double vascularization (from both left anterior descending and circumflex) – see also the fig 7.

http://dx.doi.org/10.5772/56062

Geometrical echocardiographic analysis. As already mentioned, the echocardiographic presentation of systolic restriction of the posterior mitral leaflet is typical: in presence of an inferior and/or lateral myocardial infarction, the posterior leaflet appears fixed in systole (and sometimes also in diastole), instead of the normal thickness of it and of the absence of fibrosis and/or calcification. The anterior leaflet is overlapping the posterior restricted leaflet (asymmetrical apposition), due to the deficit of a supporting surface in systole. The transthoracic exam is sufficient to identify the mechanism of mitral regurgitation and, equally important, to evaluate the degree of mitral regurgitation (Monin JL, 2005). The algorithm of evaluation of mitral valve geometry should be focused on the assessment of the triangle of coaptation and coaptation length (normally >6mm). In this specific condition there is an insufficient leaflet coaptation due to systolic restriction of the posterior leaflet, asymmetric apposition of the anterior leaflet and annular dilatation.

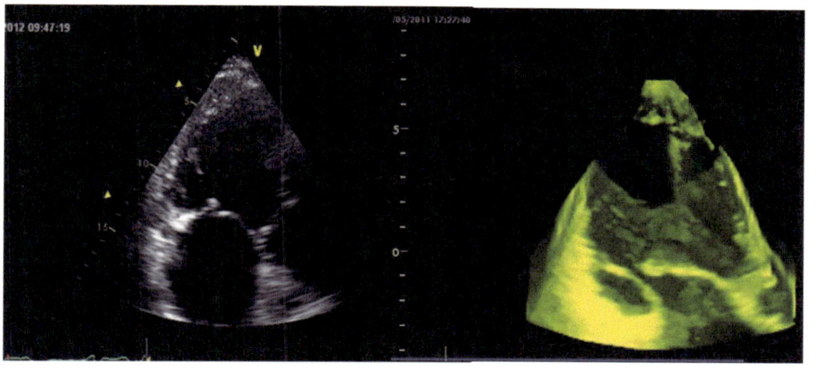

Figure 22. Restriction of posterior leaflet with typical asymmetric apposition of the anterior one (2DE and 3DE TT pictures) in a patient with inferior MI. The tip of the anterior mitral leaflet is heading towards the left atrium due to chronic loss of the systolic resistance plane.

The evaluation of the anatomical and functional reserve of the posterior mitral leaflet plays an essential role for those patients who will undergo reconstructive surgery. For example, when the posterior leaflet is too small (<1mm of length) and particularly restricted (*fixed* leaflet), it is a clear sign of reduced anatomical reserve. This key point will indicate the need of a more aggressive surgical approach where reductive annuloplasty should be associated to leaflet extension as discussed before.

Echo-surgical messages: As general rule, in coronary patients undergoing revascularization, the assessment of the severity of valve regurgitation (and so of decision to treat the regurgitation), should be done by transthoracic exam, as general anesthesia may significantly decrease the severity of regurgitation. When necessary, in the operating room, a preload and/or afterload test provides an additional estimation of the severity of mitral regurgitation (Aklog 2001, Gisbert A, 2006). Intraoperative transesophageal echocardiography is routinely performed in order to confirm the mechanism of mitral regurgitation and mainly to control the outcome of repair.

Surgical planning and management. Most of the times, the surgical technique consists in mitral annuloplasty using an undersized complete prosthetic ring or in alternative only a posterior prosthetic ring which should reduce the annular dilation especially in the region of the medial scallops (P_3). Depending on the functional and anatomical reserve of the posterior leaflet, cusp extension using a pericardial patch may be taken into consideration. The newly inserted pericardial patch should be as large as possible because, by sewing usually it remains smaller and also because it has a natural tendency to shrink overtime.

5.2. Ischemic dilatative cardiomyopathy (fig 23)

Background. This situation is the final stage of an unfavorable evolution of ischemic heart disease. Usually, in anamnesis, there are more than one myocardial infarction and a long story of percutaneous interventions and/or surgical treatments.

Mechanism. This category of patients presents the phenomenon of "mitral – ventricular mismatch". Due to progressive dilatation of the left cavity, the rightly balance between the mitral valve apparatus and the dimension of the multiinfarcted left ventricle will be lost, and in this condition, the mitral valve will become insufficient. Any tentative to repair the mitral valve has to take into consideration this aspect. More remodeled and dilated the left cavity will be, more difficult will be to accomplish the valve repair and the plasty will be less stable over time. Some elements as diameter of the LV cavity, the volumes, dilatation of the mitral annulus and migration of the papillary muscle, may be documented by a series of echocardiographic parameters. So, the remodeling of the left heart will be expressed by a series of factor as: tenting area, coaptation distance, left ventricular diameter and volume, the interpapillary distance. Some studies showed negative correlation between these parameters and the feasibility of mitral repair.

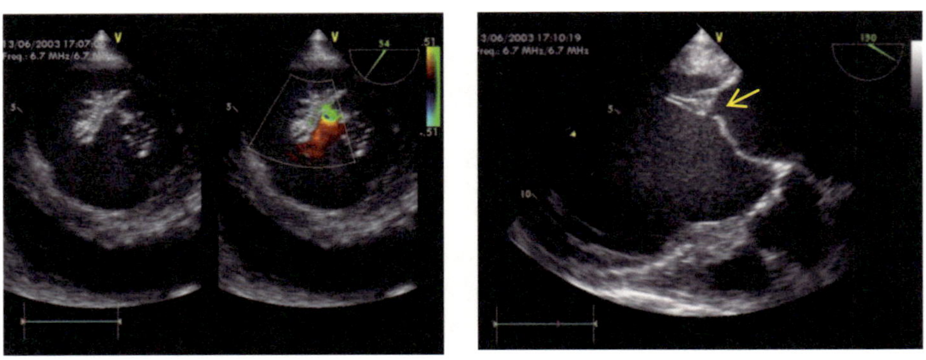

Figure 23. Ischemic dilated cardiomyopathy with chronic mitral regurgitation due to important dilatation of the LV cavity, annular dilatation and loss of leaflet coaptation (arrow). TEE transgastric short and long axis views. Notice also the systolic restriction of the posterior leaflet (right picture).

http://dx.doi.org/10.5772/56062

6. Unfavorable characteristics for mitral valve repair (table 2, fig 24)

When the global remodeling of the left ventricle is too advanced, with loss of the normal shape and important dilatation of the LV cavity, overt tethering of the mitral leaflet and important annular dilatation, the mitral valve repair may be difficult to accomplish (Troubil 2010). A remodeled, dilated ventricle, with an interpapillary muscle distance more than 20mm, is a marker of poor scenario for mitral valve repair. A left ventricular cavity remodeled and dilated with a value above 65mm for LV end diastolic diameter (EDD) and above 51mm for end systolic diameter (ESD), corresponding to an end systolic volume above 140ml, are also considered unfavorable characteristics for valve repair.

• Coaptation distance ≥ 1 cm
• Tenting area > 2,5 – 3 cm^2
• Complex jets
• Posterolateral angle > 45°
• Interpapillary muscle distance > 20 mm
• EDD > 65 mm, ESD > 51 mm (ESV > 140 mL)

EDD - end diastolic diameter,

ESD - end systolic diameter,

ESV - end systolic volume.

Table 2. Unfavorable characteristics for mitral valve repair.

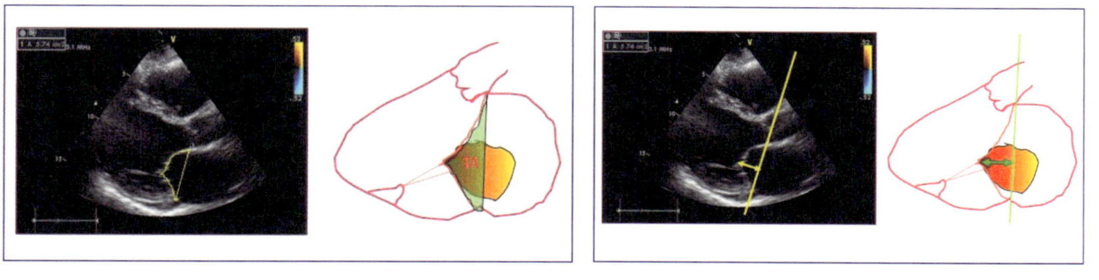

Figure 24. Assessment of the tenting area (5,74cm^2, left) and of the coaptation distance (13mm, right) in a coronary patient with chronic ischemic mitral insufficiency; both criteria suggest low probability for mitral valve repair.

Due to the deteriorated contractile status of the LV, the diminish force of closing contributes to the generation of mitral insufficiency, but this phenomenon alone is not enough. There are indeed forms of dilated cardiomyopathy with very large ventricle and severely reduced ejection fraction without an important mitral regurgitation, or even without any mitral regurgitation. Important in this situation is the impairment of the geometry at the papillary muscles level. Asymmetrical and symmetrical pattern can coexist in the same patient.

Geometrical echocardiographic analysis. These patients have a high degree of tenting in both leaflets (papillary far from each other), a very dilated annulus and a large defect of coaptation in the central part of the valve conditioning a severe mitral regurgitation, with a large vena contracta. They also present a larger area than normal of the coaptation triangle, express by a larger tenting area and a higher coaptation distance (fig 24).

Surgery. Given the seriousness of this clinical condition, the surgical management of this syndrome requires the most aggressive approach. Restrictive and undersized annuloplasty usually with a complete rigid is often combined with other surgical techniques as leaflet extension and/or papillary muscle repositioning. There are some techniques used in these situations, like re-approaching the papillary muscles with a Gore-Tex band (Hvass 2010) thus decreasing the degree of tenting or the use of an external mesh for preventing further dilatation. Even if the immediate outcome could be satisfactory medium and long term results are to be evaluated.

7. Chronic ischemic mitral regurgitation due to elongation of papillary muscle (fig 24)

Background. This type of ischemic mitral regurgitation is considered to be rare (about 2% of all cases of ischemic mitral regurgitation), belonging to the Carpantier's type II classification. Nevertheless, it is possible that this type of regurgitation is indeed more frequent and in every day practice but also underestimated. The valve leakage is, here, the result of alteration of subvalvular apparatus secondary to ischemic elongation of the papillary muscle following myocardial necrosis, chronic ischemia and mechanical stress. The papillary muscle elongation is never solitary, being an associated process in the general context of post-infarction remodeling.

Mechanism. The partially infarcted and/or ischemic posterior papillary muscle suffers a chronic remodeling with elongation that expresses itself at the level of the mitral leaflets by alteration of the coaptation triangle and valve geometry.

Geometrical echocardiographic analysis: in this specific condition there is an insufficient leaflet coaptation due to various degree of ischemic prolapse of the posterior and/or anterior mitral leaflet. Often the echocardiographic aspect is an unusual anterior leaflet prolapse or that of a prolapse of more corresponding scallops (e.g. A_2/P_2 and A_3/P_3). The papillary muscle appears elongated, triangular shaped, with the tip very close to the mitral annulus. As a consequence, the normal configuration of mitral valve, defined by the coaptation triangle, will suffer various degree of alteration, till the complete disappearance (see also fig 5, 6). An annular dilation is often associated, depending on the extension of myocardial infarction. All these elements will lead to a complex holosystolic regurgitant jet. This entity may be caused by a limited infarction at the papillary muscle level, which lead to fibrosis and elongation of the muscle. The papillary muscle will develop a thin and sharp appearance, like a thorn, and will be more hyperechogenic.

http://dx.doi.org/10.5772/56062

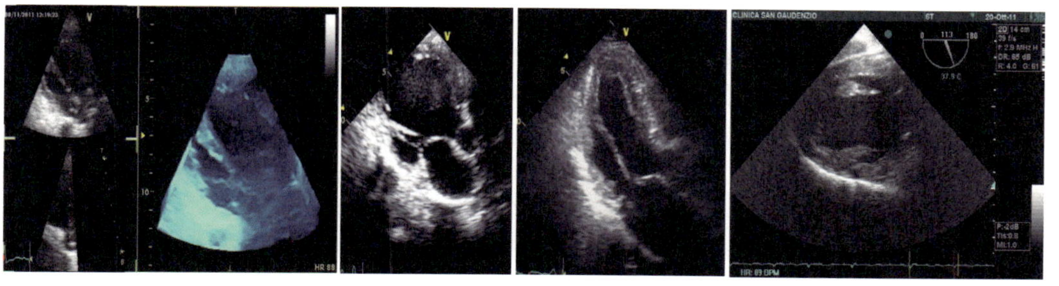

Figure 25. Several patients with chronic ischemic regurgitation and papillary muscle elongation. The papillary muscle appears elongated, thinly and sharply, like a thorn, with a hyperechogenic tip, which is very close to the mitral valve annulus plane (so called "thorny papillary muscle").

The clue of the diagnosis is the visualization of the papillary muscles, which can be done transthoracic in parasternal or apical long axis views, modified for the exposure of the papillary, or transoesophageal at 60º (bicommissural view) or transgastric view at 90º. The prolapse at the level of one scallop can coexist with the restriction of another scallop, hence the importance to visualize the entire valve prior to surgery.

Surgical planning and management: In these cases a rebuilding of the triangle of coaptation is performed by means of PTFE Gore-Tex neochords which will correct the normal mitral geometry. Depending on the intraoperative finding and surgical exposition and access, plication of the elongated papillary muscle may be performed. Annuloplasty is always performed in order to stabilize the repair.

Dyssynchrony as a cause of chronic ischemic mitral regurgitation. Due to the high prevalence of left bundle branch block in the ischemic heart disease, the assyncronism of contraction is a frequent cause of mitral regurgitation. Significant mitral regurgitation is twice more often in patients with a QRS duration longer than 130 msec. The delayed activation of the antero-lateral papillary muscle leads to a misalignment of the leaflets during systole. The resynchronization therapy has good results in this type of mitral regurgitation. The pacing wires are better attached intraoperatively, the surgeon having the possibility to choose the place without the restriction imposed by the anatomy of the cardiac veins.

On one hand, though, the currently available techniques still need validation and, on the other, the optimal therapy /combination of therapies needs clarification.

8. Conclusions

Ischemic mitral regurgitation has important prognosis implications in patients with coronary heart disease. It should not be underestimated and this underlines the need for a complete evaluation in which the 2DE and the Doppler echocardiography plays a major role, but should be interpreted specifically, in particular as regards quantification of the regurgitation.

A complete assessment of left ventricular geometry and function and of the mitral valve configuration prior to surgery may help improve patient risk stratification and better individualize the surgical strategy based on the patient's specific characteristics.

The acute ischemic mitral regurgitation is a rare mechanical complication after myocardial infarction, due to elongation, partial or complete rupture of papillary muscle but has a poor prognosis and it needs urgent diagnosis and surgery. A careful echocardiographic exam, performed in ICU, is mandatory in acute patients with myocardial infarction, focusing the attention on the presence of mitral regurgitation. In case of any suspicion of structural acute ischemic mitral regurgitation the transesophageal exam must be done, to avoid the transformation of partial rupture of papillary muscle in a complete one. The complete rupture of papillary muscle is often fatal and has to be considered a too late clinical and echocardiographic diagnosis; these patients need an emergent operation and very intensive perioperative pharmacologic and mechanical support.

From a conceptual point of view, chronic ischemic mitral regurgitation witnesses the loss of contractile myocardial tissue parallel with the presence of the post-infarction remodeling process. As known, ischemic mitral insufficiency develops on normally mitral leaflets. As the myocardial mass loss is larger, the remodeling processes and regurgitation become greater.

Recognizing the mechanism of valve incompetence is an essential point for the surgical planning and for a good result of the mitral repair. In the patient's candidates to surgery, the role of the echocardiographic exam is to identify the mechanisms of valve regurgitation and to quantify it. As noted, in most cases of chronic ischemic mitral regurgitation the mechanism is the restriction of one or both leaflets, caused by the tethering exercised by the displaced papillary muscle.

The transthoracic exam is commonly enough to clarify the mechanism of the chronic ischemic mitral regurgitation. Only patients with papillary muscle elongation may raise difficulties in diagnosis. Loss of the normal shape of the 'triangle of coaptation' is one of the key characteristics of chronic ischemic mitral regurgitation. In case of post-ischemic elongation of the papillary muscle, the clue of the diagnosis is obtained by looking not only to the mitral valve, but by focusing the exam on the papillary muscles, particularly when the patient presents a deformation of the 'coaptation triangle'. In patients with type II° Carpentier's classifications (elongated papillary muscle and leaflets prolapse), alongside of ring annuloplasty use of PTFE Gore-Tex chordae is often required.

In patients with chronic ischemic mitral insufficiency the echocardiography may identify two different patterns of post infarction remodeling: a *limited* process of post infarction remodeling and an *extensive* one. The mitral repair is usually more challenging in patients with extensive pattern of post infarction remodeling, where, due to left heart cavity enlargement a phenomenon of "mitral valve – LV chamber mismatch" is present.

Although the mechanisms of ischemic mitral regurgitation are often complex, currently, undersized annuloplasty is considered the standard approach to reducing mitral insufficiency. Unfortunately this technique does not resolve the real mechanism of disease, the remodeled and sphericalized left ventricle. By this technique the persistence of ischemic mitral regurgitation is considered to range between 10 to 20% of the cases, and, at five years of follow up, half of the patient may develop recurrence.

Thus, in advanced stage of left ventricular post infarction remodeling with over dilatation and important mitral valve tethering, the ring annuloplasty has to be completed with leaflet extension. This approach seems coherent with the mechanism of mitral regurgitation, with the echocardiographic data and with the concept of "mitral valve – LV chamber mismatch".

The major challenge for cardiologists and surgeons is how to integrate data from different imaging techniques that assess mitral valve geometry and left ventricular size, geometry, function and potential functional recovery. This in order to tailor and optimize the surgical approach to patients with chronic ischemic mitral regurgitation.

Even today, we have no reliable predictors of recurrent and persistent mitral regurgitation. However, the surgical treatment of ischemic mitral insufficiency continues to evolve and new methods addressing ventricular structures are being introduced: left ventricular restoration, papillary muscle's relocation, sling, imbrication or reapproximation, chordal cutting or translocation. Despite remarkable progress in reparative surgery, further investigation is still necessary to find the best approach to treat ischemic mitral regurgitation.

Author details

Gheorghe Cerin[1], Adrian Bogdan Popa[1], Razvan Ticulescu[2] and Marco Diena[1]

*Address all correspondence to: gheorghe.cerin@gmail.com

1 The Cardioteam Foundation, Cardiac Surgery Dpt, San Gaudenzio Clinic, Novara, Italy

2 Cardiac Surgery Dpt, The 'Monza' Hospital, Bucharest, Romania

References

[1] "Kirklin/Barratt-Boyes Cardiac Surgery": Nicholas T. Kouchoukos, Eugene H. Blackstone, Frank L. Hanley, James K. Kirklin. 4Th edition, Publisher: Saunders; 4th Revised edition

[2] Popa B A, Diena M, Cerin G, Lanzillo G., Tesler UF.Severe Post-Ischemic Elongation of the Anterior Papillary Muscle. An Unusual Cause of Mitral Insufficiency in a 75-Year-Old Man; Tex Heart Inst J. (2007); 34(2): 222-224.

[3] Carpentier's Reconstructive Valve Surgery, Alain Carpentier, David Adams, Farzan-Filsoufi, Saunders, 2010.

[4] Carpentier A. Cardiac valve surgery:the French correction. J ThoracCardiovascSurg. 1983; 86: 323–337.

[5] Cerin G, Popa BA, Benea D, Lanzillo G, Karazanishvili L, Casati V, Popa A, Novelli E, Renzi L, Diena M. The triangle of coaptation: a new concept to enhance mitral valve repair through reshaping the native geometry. Circ. 2010; 122: e115. Published online before print June 14, 2010, doi: 10.1161/ CIRCULATION AHA.110.192774.

[6] Clements SD Jr, Story WE, Hurst JW, Craver JM, Jones EL. Ruptured papillary muscle, a complication of myocardial infarction: clinical presentation, diagnosis, and treatment. ClinCardiol. (1985);8(2), 93-103.

[7] Cohn LH, Rizzo R J, Adams DH et al. The effect of pathophysiology on the surgical treatment of ischemic mitral regurgitation: operative and late risks of repair versus replacement. Eur J CardioThoracSurg (1995); 9: 568-74.

[8] Dagum P, Timek TA, Green, G R, et al. Coordinate-free analysis of mitral valve dynamics in normal and ischemic hearts. Circulation (2000) 102(19 Suppl 3):III62-9.

[9] De Varennes B, Chaturvedi R, Sidhu S, Côté A. Li Pi Shan W, Goyer C, Hatzakorzian R, Buithieu J, Sniderman A Initial Results of Posterior Leaflet Extension for Severe Type IIIb Ischemic Mitral Regurgitation Circulation. (2009) 2;119(21):2837-43.

[10] Dobre M, Koul B, Rojer A. Anatomic and physiologic correction of the restricted posterior mitral leaflet motion in chronic ischemic mitral regurgitation. J Thor CardiovascSurg. (2000); 120 (2): 409-411.

[11] Estes EH Jr., Dalton FM, Entman ML, Dixon HB II, Hackel DB. The anatomy and blood supply of the papillary muscles of the left ventricle. AmHeart J 1966; 71(3): 356-362.

[12] Fattouch K, Guccione F, Sampognaro R, Panzarella G, Corrado E, Navarra E, Calvaruso D, Ruvolo G. POINT: Efficacy of adding mitral valve restrictive annuloplasty to coronary artery bypass grafting in patients with moderate ischemic mitral valve regurgitation: a randomized trial. J Thorac Cardiovasc Surg. 2009;138:278–85.

[13] Fattouch K, Sampognaro R, Speziale G, Salardino M, Novo G, Caruso M, Novo S, Ruvolo G. Impact of moderate ischemic mitral regurgitation after isolated coronary artery bypass grafting. AnnThoracSurg. 2010;90:1187–94.

[14] Cerin, G, Popa, B A, &Diena, M. The Degenerative Mitral Valve Regurgitation: From Geometrical Echocardiographic Concepts to Successful Surgical Repair; Echocardiography- In Specific Diseases, (2012). 978-9-53307-977-6DOI:

[15] G Cerin, M Diena, G Lanzillo, S Casalino, A Zito, D Benea, U Filippo Tesler. Degenerative mitral regurgitation - surgical and echocardiographic consideration for repair. Romanian Journal of Cardiovascular Surgery, 5 (3), pp. 131-39, 2006.

[16] Aklog L, Filsoufi F, Flores KQ, et al: Does coronary artery bypass grafting alone correct moderate ischemic mitral regurgitation? Circulation 2001;104(12 Suppl 1):I68-I75.

[17] Gisbert A, Soulière V, Denault AY, Bouchard D, Couture P, Pellerin M, Carrier M, Levesque S, Ducharme A, Basmadjian AJ. Dynamic quantitative echocardiographic evaluation of mitral regurgitation in the operating department. J AmSocEchocardiogr. 2006 Feb;19(2):140-6.

[18] Green GR, Dagum P, Glasson JR, Daughters GT, Bolger AF, Foppiano LE, Berry GJ, Ingels NB Jr, Miller DC; Mitral annular dilatation and papillary muscle dislocation without mitral regurgitation in sheep. Circulation. 1999 Nov 9;100(19 Suppl):II95-102.

[19] Grigioni F, Enriquez-Sarano, M, Zehr, K. J, Bailey, K. R, & Tajik, A. J. Ischemic mitral regurgitation: long-term outcome and prognostic implications with quantitative Doppler assessment. Circ. (2001). , 103, 1759-1764.

[20] Grossi EA, Goldberg JD, LaPietra A, Ye X, Zakow P, Sussman M, Delianides J, Culliford AT, Esposito RA, Ribakove GH, Galloway AC, Colvin SB. Ischemic mitral valve reconstruction and replacement: comparison of long-term survival and complications. J ThoracCardiovascSurg. 2001; 122: 1107–1124.

[21] Muresian, H. (2009). The Clinical Anatomy of The Coronary Arteries. An Anatomical Study on Human Heart Specimens. Edited by H. Muresian. Ed. Enciclopedica isbn: 978-973-45-0581-4.

[22] Hvass, U. Joudinaud T The papillary muscle sling for ischemic mitral regurgitation; J Th Cardiovascular Surgery February (2010). , 139(2), 418-423.

[23] Jeroen, J. Bax; Jerry Braun; Soeresh T. Somer, Robert Klautz, Eduard R. Holman, Michel I.M. Versteegh, Eric Boersm, MSc; Martin J. Schalij, Ernst E. van der Wall, Robert A. Dion Restrictive Annuloplasty and Coronary Revascularization in Ischemic Mitral Regurgitation Results in Reverse Left Ventricular Remodeling. Circulation. (2004). suppl II]: II-II-108., 103.

[24] Lamas GA, Mitchell GF, Flaker GC, Smith Jr SC, Gersh BJ, Basta L, Movè L, Braunwald E, Pfeffer MA. Clinical significance of mitral regurgitation after acute myocardial infarction. Survival and Ventricular Enlargement. Circulation 1997; 96:827-833. doi: 10.1161/01.CIR.96.3.827.

[25] Langer F, Rodriguez F, Cheng A, Ortiz S, Nguyen T C, Zasio M K, BA, Liang D, Daughters G T, Ingels N B, D. Miller C. Posterior mitral leaflet extension: An adjunctive repair option for ischemic mitral regurgitation? J Thor CardiovascSurg 2006;131:868-877 .

[26] Levine RA, Hung J, Otsuji Y, Messas E, Liel-Cohen N, Nathan N, Handschumacher MD, Guerrero JL, He S, Yoganathan AP, Vlahakes GJ. Mechanisticinsightsintofunctional mitral regurgitation. Current Cardiol Reports 2002; 4(2):125-129.

[27] Loisance DY, Deleuze PH, Hillion ML, Cachera JP: Are there indications for reconstructive surgery in severe mitral regurgitation after acute myocardial infarction? Eur J CardiothoracSurg 1990; 4:394-97.

[28] Troubil, M, Lonsky, V, &Gwozdziewicz, M. V. Bruk Persistent and recurrent ischemic mitral regurgitation; Biomed Pap Med FacUnivPalacky Olomouc Czech Rep. (2010). Jun; 154(2), 141-145.

[29] Magne, J, Sénéchal, M, &Dumesnil, J. G. Pibarot P; Ischemic mitral regurgitation: a complex multifaceted disease. Cardiology. 2009;doi:Epub (2008). Aug 30, 112(4), 6 244-59.

[30] McGee EC, Gillinov AM, Blackstone EH, Lytle BW, McCarthy PM, Cosgrove DM. Recurrent mitral regurgitation after annuloplasty for functional ischemic mitral regurgitation. J ThoracCardiovascSurg. 2004; 128: 916–924.

[31] Messas E, Guerrero JL, Handschumacher MD, Chow C-M, Sullivan S, Yoganathan A P, Levine RA Chordal cutting: a new therapeutic approach for ischemic mitral regurgitation. Circulation 2001;104(16):1958-1963; doi: 10.1161/hc4201.097135.

[32] Mitesh V. Badiwala, SubodhVerma and VivekRao; Surgical Management of Ischemic Mitral Regurgitation. Circulation 2009; 120; 1287-1293; doi: 10.1161/CIRCULATIONAHA.108.836627.

[33] Monin J-L, Dehant P, Roiron C, Monchi M, Tabet J-Y, Clerc P, Fernandez G, Houel R, Garot J, Chauvel C, Gueret P; Functional assessment of mitral regurgitation by transthoracic echocardiography using standardized imaging planes: diagnostic accuracy and outcome implications. J AmCollCardiol 2005; 46(2):302-309. doi:10.1016/j.jacc.2005.03.064.

[34] Otto, C. (2012). The Practice of Clinical Echocardiography, 4th Edition, W. B. Saunders Company, 978-1-43772-765-4Philadelphia, USA.

[35] Patrick Klein. Jerry Braun, Eduard R. Holman, Michel I.M. Versteegh, Harriette F. Verwey, Robert A.E. Dion, Jeroen J. Bax and Robert J.M. Klautz; Management of mitral regurgitation during left ventricular reconstruction for Iischemic heart failure European Journal of Cardio-Thoracic Surgery (2012). doi:10.1016/j.ejcts.2011.04.035, 41(2012), 74-81.

[36] Zegdi R, Khabbaz Z, Chauvaud S, Latremouille C, Fabiani J-N, &Deloche A. Posterior Leaflet Extension With an Autologous Pericardial Patch in Rheumatic Mitral Insufficiency Ann ThoracSurg (2007), 84, 1043-4.

[37] Rankin JS, Feneley MP, Hickey M St J, Muhlbaier LH, Wechsler AS, Floyd RA, Skelton TN, Califf RM, Lowe JE et al. A clinical comparison of mitral valve repair versus valve replacement in ischemic mitral regurgitation. J ThoracCardiovascSurg 1988;95:165–77.

[38] Stevenson L. W. Grover-McKay M, Brucken RC, et al: Effects of afterload reduction (diuretics and vasodilators) on left ventricular volume and mitral regurgitation in se-

vere congestive heart failure secondary to ischemic or idiopathic dilated cardiomyopathy. Am J Cardiol (1987); 60, 654-658.

[39] Tcheng JE, Jackman JD Jr, Nelson CL, gardner LH, Rankin JS, Califf RM, Stack RS: Outcome of patients sustaining acute ischemic mitral regurgitation during myocardial infarction. AnnIntMed 1992; 117:18-24.

[40] Timek TA, Lai DT, Tibayan F, Liang D, Daughters GT, Dagum P, Zasio MK, Lo S, Hastie T, Ingles NB Jr, Miller DC. Ischemia in three left ventricular regions: Insights into the pathogenesis of acute ischemic mitral regurgitation. J ThoracCardiovascSurg 2003;125(3):559-569.

[41] Tesler, U F, Cerin, G, & Novelli, E. Anamaria Popa, M Diena. Evolution of Surgical-Techniques for Mitral Valve Repair. Tex HeartInst J. (2009). PMCID: PMC2763455, 36(5), 438-440.

[42] Zoghbi WA, Enriquez-Sarano M, Foster E, et al. Recommendations for the evaluation of the severity of native valvular regurgitation with two-dimensional and Doppler echocardiography. J AmSoc of Echocardiography. 2003;16:777–80.

[43] Hashim SW, Yousuef SJ, Ayash B, Rousou AJ, Ragnarsson S, ColazzoS,Geirson A, Pseudoprolpase of the anterior leaflet in chronic mitral ischemic regurgitation: Identification and repair. J ThoraciccardiovascSurg 2012, 143; S33-S37.

Chapter 5

Real-Time 3D Echocardiography in Percutaneous Balloon Mitral Valvuloplasty

Mark A. Navarro, Michael Kim and
Ernesto E. Salcedo

Additional information is available at the end of the chapter

http://dx.doi.org/10.5772/56433

1. Introduction

Since Dr Kanji Inoue introduced the Inoue balloon catheter in 1984, percutaneous balloon valvuloplasty (PBMV) has become the treatment of choice for patients with symptomatic mitral valve stenosis and favorable valve morphology. PBMV is the preferred treatment for mitral stenosis as it is less invasive and provides longer-lasting results than closed commissurotomy. 1 PMBV is not suited for patients with mitral stenosis due to severe annular calcification or markedly degenerated valves. PBMV can be performed either an in antegrade fashion through a transseptal puncture or retrograde from the aorta to the mitral valve. Serial balloon dilations of the mitral valve using the self-centering Inoue balloon catheter (or alternatively, a standard valvuloplasty balloon catheter) are performed to physically split the mitral valve leaflet commissures and subsequently improve leaflet motion and hemodynamics. In successful cases, percutaneous balloon mitral valvuloplasty typically doubles the mitral valve area and decreases the mitral valve gradient by half. Splitting of the commissures is the principle mechanism that leads to improvement of hemodynamics and patient symptomatology.

The anatomy of the mitral valve is complex, and echocardiographic imaging plays a critical role in both the diagnosis and guidance of management of patients with mitral stenosis. Although Doppler hemodynamics and 2D transthoracic echocardiography are a mainstay in the echocardiographic assessment of mitral stenosis (Figure 1), real-time three-dimensional echocardiography (RT3DE) is an emerging imaging tool for not only the diagnosis of mitral stenosis (Figure 2), but also for the guidance of percutaneous balloon mitral valvuloplasty procedures in the catheterization laboratory.

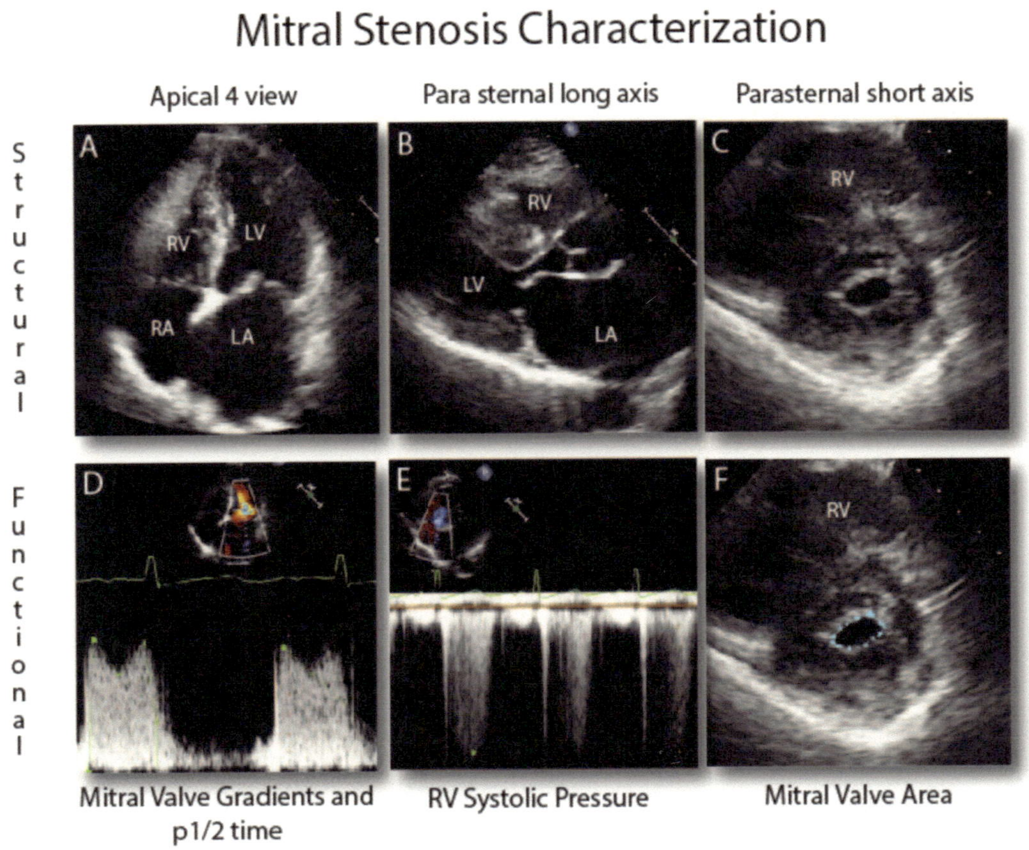

RV: right ventricle; LV: left ventricle; RA: right atrium; LA: left atrium

Figure 1. Two dimensional and Doppler echocardiography in mitral stenosis. Traditionally 2D echocardiography has provided structural information regarding the morphology of the mitral valve in mitral stenosis. In addition chamber size, and ventricular function is assessed by echocardiography. Doppler methods provide hemodynamic functional information regarding the mitral valve in mitral stenosis. Peak and mean mitral valve gradients, pressure half time derived mitral valve area and systolic pulmonary pressure are usually recorded in these patients.

2. Diagnosis

Diagnosis of mitral valve stenosis commonly involves the use of 2D transthoracic echocardiography (2DE) to assess the severity of mitral disease, including mitral leaflet mobility, thickening, calcification and sub-valvular stenosis; as well as to exclude any contraindications to treatment, such us left atrial thrombus or significant mitral regurgitation.

Normal mitral valve area (MVA) is approximately 4-6 cm^2. Patients with symptomatic mitral stenosis typically have a valve area of less than 2.0 cm^2 and have severe mitral stenosis if the valve area is less than 1.0 cm^2.[2] (Figure 3) The narrowing of the mitral orifice creates a left atrioventricular pressure gradient (the hemodynamic hallmark of mitral stenosis), which in a

http://dx.doi.org/10.5772/56433

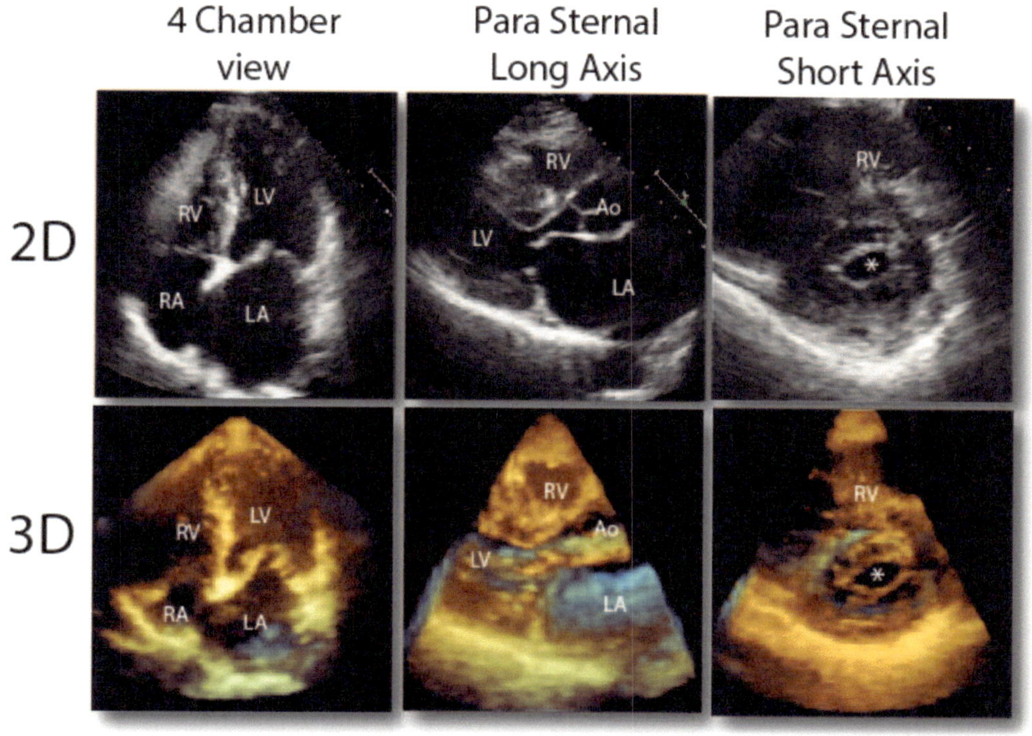

RV: right ventricle; LV: left ventricle; RA: right atrium; LA: left atrium; Ao: Aorta

Figure 2. Comparison of 2D and 3D transthoracic echocardiography in mitral stenosis. The most useful views to evaluate patients with mitral stenosis include the apical 4 chamber view as well as the parasternal long and short axis views. This figure illustrates the added value of 3D imaging in better characterizing the mitral valve apparatus. The third dimension increases the anatomic detail of the leaflets, commissures and subvalvular tissue.

normal functioning mitral valve is near zero. In the setting of hemodynamically significant mitral stenosis, patients can present with a constellation of symptoms that may include dyspnea, orthopnea, paroxysmal nocturnal dyspnea, lower extremity edema, poor exercise tolerance and/or palpitations.

3. Modalities used to evaluate the mitral valve

Various echocardiographic techniques can be used to measure mitral valve area, including pressure half-time (PHT), planimetry, continuity equation and proximal iso-velocity surface area (PISA). Each method has its own advantages and disadvantages.

Planimetry has shown to be more accurate when measuring MVA post PBMV compared to PHT, PISA or the continuity equation method.[3],[4] Planimetry involves the direct measurement of the mitral valve orifice and has correlated well with invasive anatomic measurement.[1] This method requires a considerable amount of expertise for reliability.

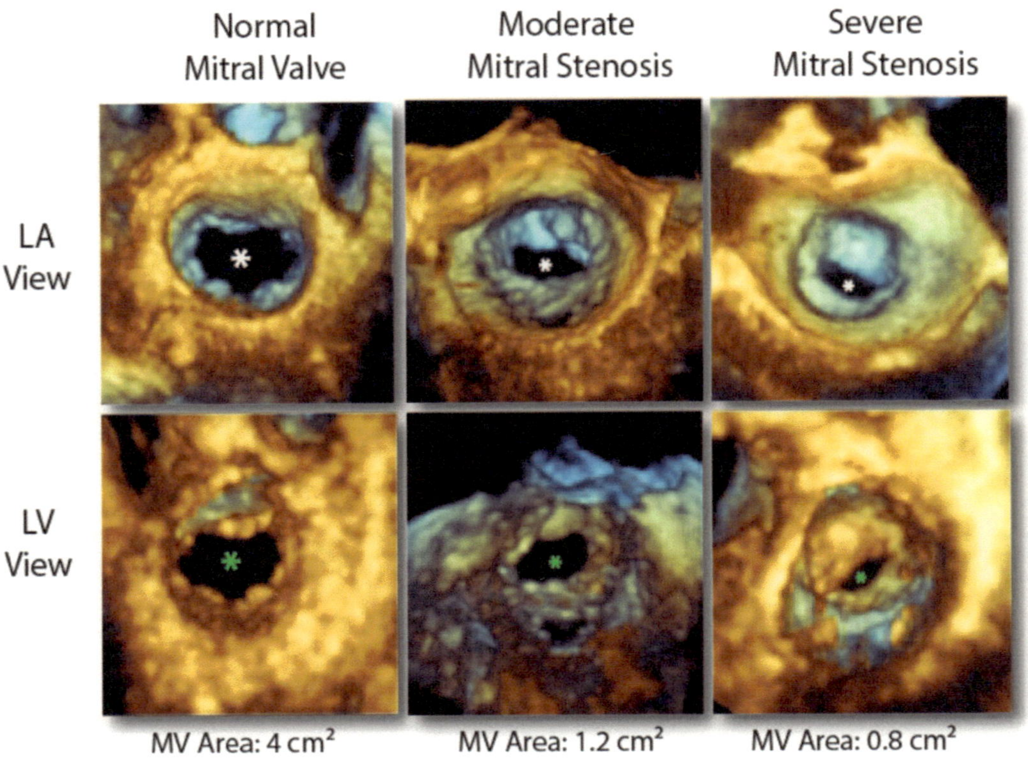

Figure 3. Normal mitral valve compared to mitral valves with moderate and severe mitral stenosis.The mitral valve orifice is seen from the left atrial side (LA view-white asterisk) and the left ventricular side (LV View- green asterisk) in a patient with a normal mitral valve (valve area 4cm^2, a patient with moderate mitral stenosis (valve area of 1.2 cm$^{2)}$, and in a patient with severe mitral stenosis (valve area of 0.8 cm^2).

The PHT method is easily performed, but is influenced by other concomitant valvular disease, such as aortic or mitral regurgitation, or by the dynamic hemodynamics seen post-PBMV.[4],[6],[7] In contrast, planimetry is not affected by hemodynamic variability, but is difficult because it requires technically challenging imaging views of the mitral orifice.

The PISA method requires many different imaging planes and variables to accurately calculate MVA and thus is very laborious. It can be however, used in the presence of mitral regurgitation dynamic flow changes.[7]

The continuity equation also involves the measurements of many variables, including size of the left ventricular outflow tract and mitral annulus. It also cannot be used in patients with atrial fibrillation or significant aortic or mitral regurgitation.

Planimetry has become the most reliable method for calculating mitral valve area and has been compared to the invasively derived Gorlin's formula, which by some is considered the gold standard for mitral valve area calculation.[2] However, real-time 3D echocardiography (RT3DE) may be a more accurate and feasible method for calculating MVA in patients being evaluated for PBMV.[6] Planimetry with 2DE relies on good echocardiographic technique and imaging windows in the parasternal short-axis plane to directly measure the mitral valve orifice. In contrast, RT3DE is not limited to a specific imaging plane and can image the mitral valve in several different planes, allowing for a recreation of a 3D image for precise tracing of the mitral valve orifice.(Figure 4) Even though poor imaging windows can affect both 2D and 3D echocardiography, RT3DE has been less affected by poor imaging windows compared to 2D.[8],[9] Real-time 3D echocardiography has been shown to be more accurate and reliable than 2DE planimetry for assessing MVA, severity of commissural fusion and extent of sub-valvular disease.[8],[10] Real-time 3D echocardiography has also been shown to provide a more accurate and reliable MVA measurement in inexperienced echocardiographers using RT3DE compared to 2D echocardiography and nominally affected by mitral valve morphology and post-PBMV hemodynamic changes.[6],[8],[10]-[11]

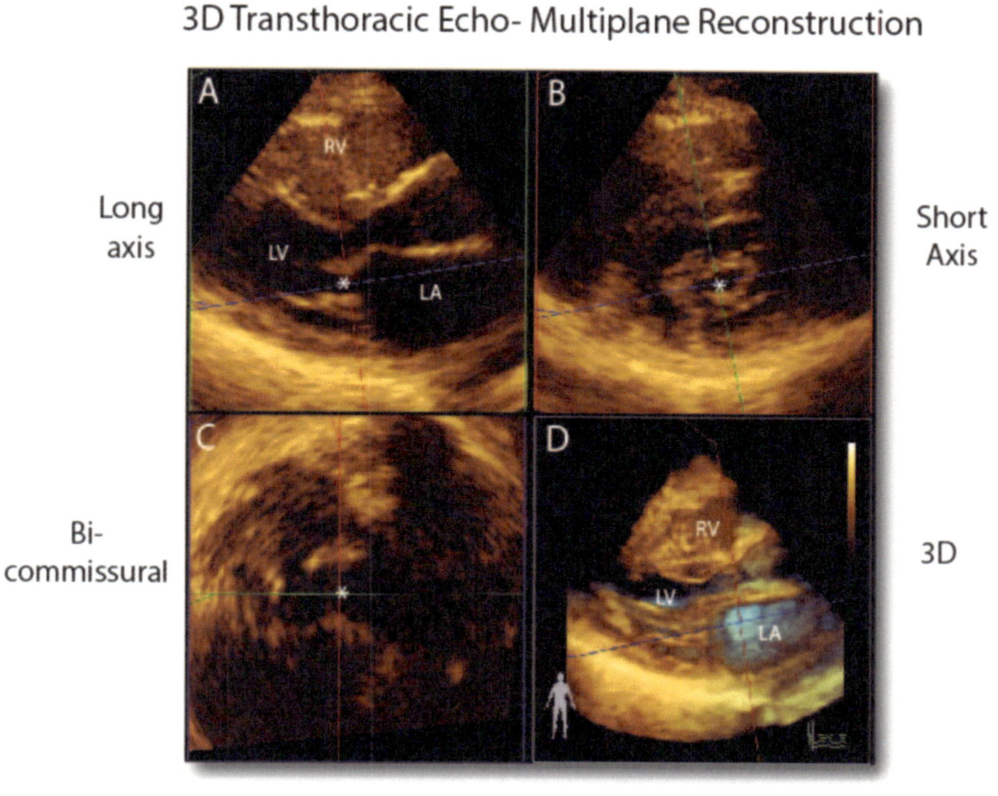

The asterisks represent the mitral valve orifice from each of the 3 orthogonal planes. RV: right ventricle; LV: left ventricle; RA: right atrium; LA: left atrium

Figure 4. Multiplane reconstruction of the mitral valve apparatus in mitral stenosis. 3D echocardiography can be presented in a volume rendition form (panel D) or in a simultaneous multiplane rendition (panels A, B and C). From the long axis plane (panel A) one can choose the tips of the leaflets to obtain the true minimal mitral valve orifice area, as depicted in panel B. Panel C represents an orthogonal view at the bi-commissural level, a view that is not obtainable from 2D echo alone.

4. Patient selection

Favorable patients for percutaneous balloon mitral valvuloplasty are typically evaluated through calculation of the echocardiographic Wilkin's score (Figure 5). It is the most widely used prognostic score to determine a favorable PBMV outcome. It is derived non-invasively by echocardiography using four variables, valve leaflet mobility, thickening, calcification and degree of sub-valvular thickening. The Wilkin's score assigns a value from 1 to 4 for each category, with a higher value indicating more extensive disease. A patient is considered a good candidate for PBMV if they have a total score of ≤ 8 and the absence of severe mitral regurgitation. An optimal patient is associated with a high level of procedural success and low complication rate. Patients with scores > 8 have an increased risk for adverse outcomes and should be considered for surgical management.[12] However, even in unfavorable candidates percutaneous balloon valvuloplasty is often still the first treatment of choice in experienced centers.

Grade	Mobility	Thickening	Calcification	Subvalvular disease
1	Highly mobile with only leaflet tips restricted	Leaflets near normal in thickness (4-5mm)	A single area of increased echo brightness	Minimal thickening just below the mitral leaflets
2	Leaflet mid portions and base portions have normal mobility	Midleaflets normal, considerable thickening of margins (5-8mm)	Scattered areas of brightness confined to leaflet margins	Thickening of chordal structures extending to one of the chordal length
3	Valve continues to move forward in diastole, mainly from the base	Thickening extending through the entire leaflets (5-8mm)	Brightness extending into the mid portions of the leaflets	Thickening extended to distal third of the chords
4	No or minimal forward movement of the leaflets in diastole	Considerable thickening of all leaflet tissue ("/>8-10mm)	Extensive brightness throughout much of the leaflet tissue	Extensive thickening and shortening of all chordal structures extending down to the papillary muscle

Adapted from Wilkins et al.[12]

Table 1. Mitral Valve Anatomy Scoring Using the Wilkin's Score

Iung and Cormier also developed a scoring system to evaluate mitral valve anatomy in a less complex way. In addition, the Cormier scoring system also factors in chordae length, a feature not included in the more traditional Wilkins score. Interestingly, however, neither the Wilkins or Cormier scoring systems address the issue of commissure disease, such as fusion and extent of calcification. Inadequate leaflet splitting and the development of mitral regurgitation can be related to severe commissural disease.[14]-[16] Identifying the degree of commissural disease can help to predict poor patient outcomes. Because of the potential importance of commissural disease in PBMV outcomes, there is interest in incorporating this variable into a new, RT3DE-derived mitral stenosis scoring system.[9]

http://dx.doi.org/10.5772/56433

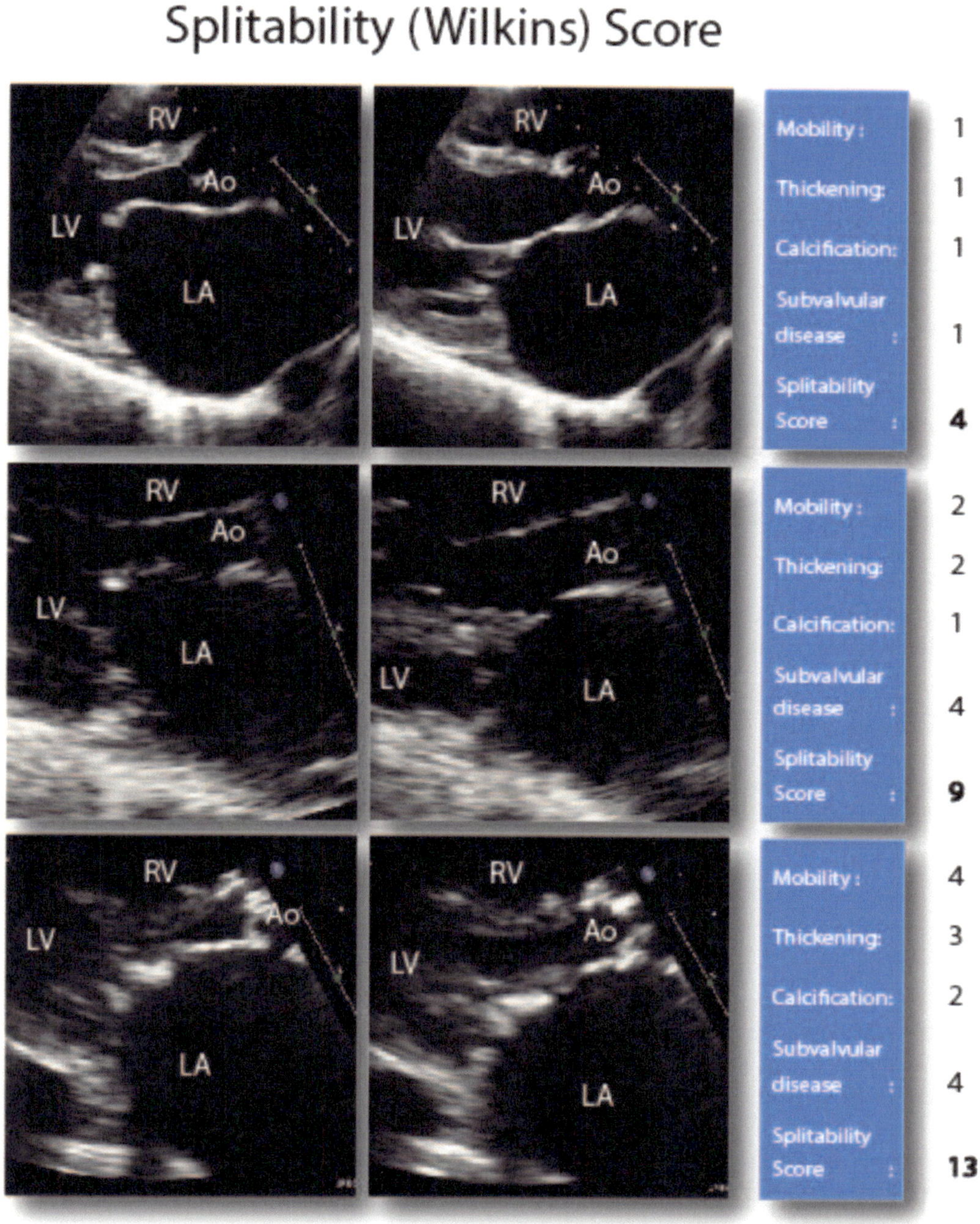

RV: right ventricle; LV: left ventricle; RA: right atrium; LA: left atrium; Ao: Aorta

Figure 5. Splitability scores obtained in three patients with mitral stenosis. Diastolic frames are depicted to the left and systolic frames to the right. The upper panels are from a patient with a Splitability score of 4, which would make him a good balloon valvuloplasty candidate. The middle panels are from a patient with a score of 9 which would make him a borderline candidate for valvuloplasty. The lower panels are from a poor candidate for balloon valvuloplasty with a score of 13.

Echocardiographic Grade	Mitral valve anatomy
1	Pliable non-calcified anterior mitral leaflet and mild subvalvular disease (i.e., thin chordae 10mm long)
2	Pliable non-calcified anterior mitral leaflet and severe subvalvular disease (i.e., thickened chordae < 10mm long)
3	Calcification of mitral valve of any extent, as assessed by fluoroscopy, whatever state of the subvalvular apparatus.

Adapted by Iung B et al.[13]

Table 2. Cormier Score

When compared to 2DE, real-time 3D echocardiography allows for superior visualization of the mitral valve and sub-valvular anatomy. (Figure 2) Specifically, real-time 3D echocardiography allows for better resolution of mitral leaflet thickening and annular calcification and enhanced anatomic detail of chordal thickening and separation.[9] Commissural separation, a key determinate of PBMV success is also better assessed by RT3DE.[10] Finally, leaflet calcification, including distribution of calcium is better visualized with RT3DE. This is important because leaflet calcification is a strong predictor of commissural splitting. The presence of calcification also can help predict adverse outcomes such as embolic stroke or conduction abnormalities.[9]

1. Persistent left atrial or left atrial appendage thrombus
2. Severe mitral regurgitation
3. Massive or bicommissural calcification
4. Severe concomitant aortic valve or severe tricuspid regurgitation or stenosis
5. Severe concomitant coronary artery disease requiring bypass surgery

Adapted from ACC/AHA 2006 Guidelines for the management of valvular heart disease.[17]

Table 3. Contraindications to percutaneous balloon mitral valvuloplasty

Contraindications to PBMV are listed in Table 3. However, with the advancement of technique and imaging, even "unfavorable" candidates are often considered for PBMV as first line treatment in experienced centers. Other patient factors such as age, presence of severe pulmonary hypertension, atrial arrhythmia, history of prior commissurotomy, smaller valve area, presence of mitral regurgitation, NYHA class IV and surgical risk help determine those patients best suited for PBMV.[13],[18],[19]

5. Immediate and late results

The successful splitting of the commissures is the primary determinant of procedural success. A mitral valve gradient that decreases to 50% pre-PBMV gradient and a mitral valve area that

http://dx.doi.org/10.5772/56433

roughly increases by 100% or > 1.5cm² without significant mitral regurgitation are hemodynamic criteria used to gauge success.[20] Other, often unmeasured variables such as exercise capacity, pulmonary pressures, left atrial pressure and cardiac output also increase respectively.

At the time of the procedure), we rely heavily on echo evidence of bicommissural splitting, which is best seen with RT 3D TEE (Figure 6). The reason for this is that patients undergoing PMBV are usually under general anesthesia, or heavily sedated, which dramatically impacts the hemodynamics through the valve. An anatomic endpoint, as opposed to a hemodynamic endpoint, is what is generally used to assess the efficacy of the PMBV.

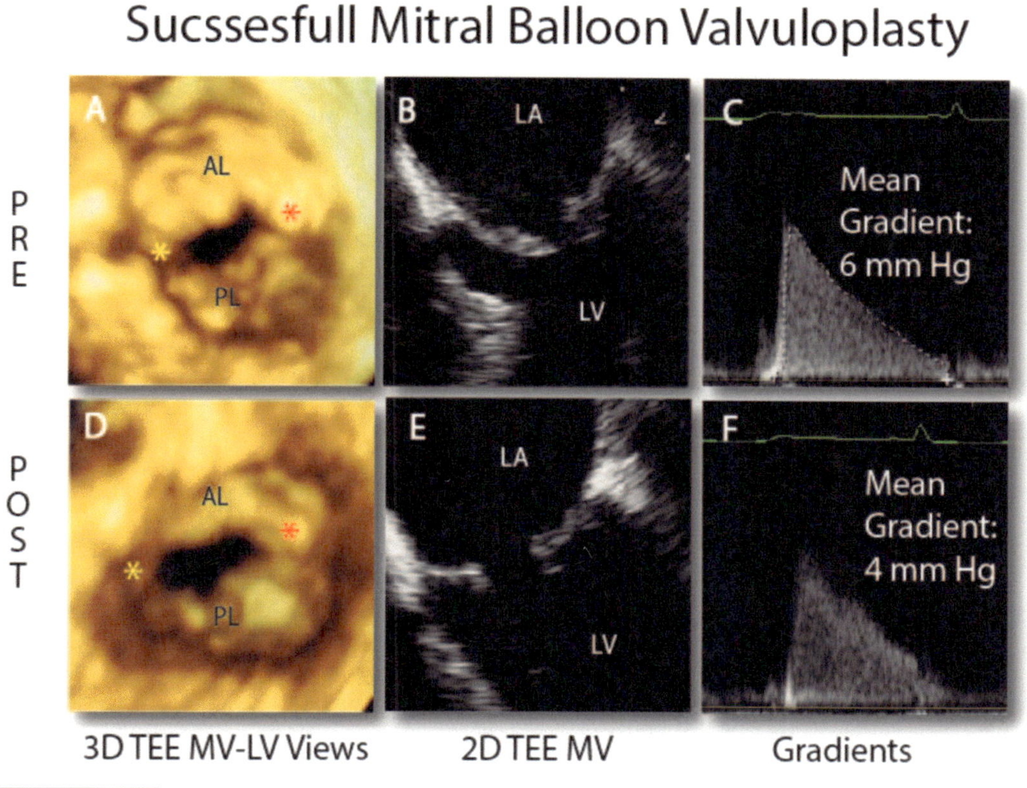

Yellow asterisk: lateral commissure; red asterisk: medial commissure.

Figure 6. Panels A and D depict the mitral valve orifice as seen from the LV. Note the commissural fusion and the small mitral orifice in the pre procedure image (Panel A). In panel D, were the commissures are now split and the arealof the mitral orifice has increased. Panels B and E illustrate the 2D TEE views of the mitral valve pre and post procedure. Note the increased leaflet distance post procedure. Panels C and F illustrate the transmitral Doppler gradients pre and post procedure. The pre-procedure gradients had already diminished under general anesthesia and the post procedure gradients showed only a mild drop despite good bi-commissural splitting. This is not uncommon to see in the immediate post procedure studies and is probably related to decreased left atrial compliance, therefore to gage procedural success; we rely mostly on the 3D visualization of the mitral orifice size and commissural splitting.

Late re-stenosis is defined as a valve area < 1.5cm^2 or a > 50% decrease of initial increase in valve area post- PBMV.[21] Patients with optimal anatomy (Wilkin's score ≤ 8) have a re-stenosis rate nearly 15% less for the same time frame of those with non-optimal anatomy.[20]

Favorable long-term results are directly correlated to desirable baseline valve anatomy and good immediate results of PBMV.[18] Favorable patients with Wilkin's scores < 8 have less re-stenosis as those with scores > 8.[20],[22] In addition, several clinical factors have been shown to influence late PBMV results: NYHA functional class III-IV, age ≥ 70 years atrial fibrillation, and suboptimal valve morphology after the procedure.[18] Unsuccessful balloon commissurotomy (Figure 7) and incomplete commissural splitting is associated with a higher post-procedure mitral gradient and smaller post-PBMV valve area.

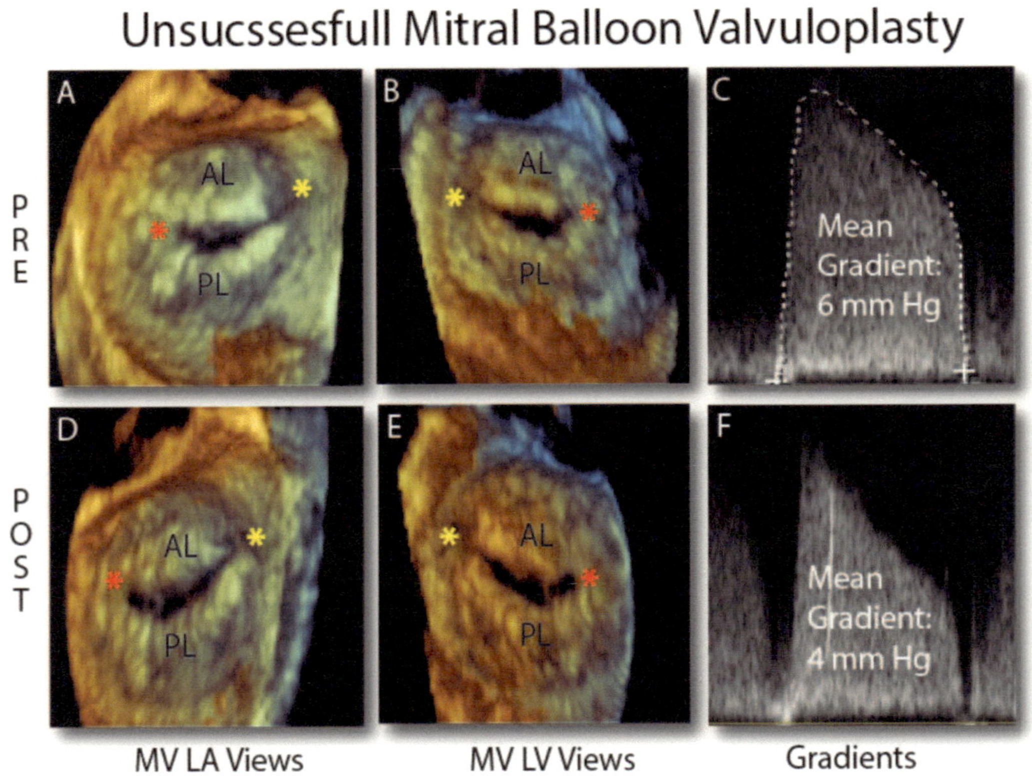

Yellow asterisk: lateral commissure; red asterisk: medial commissure
AL: anterior leaflet; PL: posterior leaflet

Figure 7. Panels A and D depict the mitral valve orifice as seen from the LA. Note the commissural fusion and the small mitral orifice in the pre procedure image. In panel D, post procedure, the commissures are not splitted and the area of the mitral orifice has not increased. Panels B and E illustrate the views of the mitral valve from the left ventricle with similar findings.. Panels C and F illustrate the transmitral Doppler gradients pre and post procedure showing no significant drop in mean transmitral pressures

http://dx.doi.org/10.5772/56433

Event-free survival; Table 4, has been shown to be as high as 90% in 5 years or longer after the procedure.[23]

Study	(n) patients	Age (yrs)	Follow-up (yrs)	Event –free Survival (%)
Fawzy et al.[24]	520	31	17	31±
Iung et al.[18]	1024	49	10	56±
Palacios et al.[26]	879	55	12	33±
Ben-Farhat et al.[25]	654	34	10	72±
Song et al.[23]	402	44	9	90*
Fawzy [28]	547	31	10	88
Cohen [27]	136	59	5	51*

*Survival without intervention

± Survival without intervention in NYHA I or II

Table 4. Event Free Survival

6. Procedural complications

Rates of success of PBMV can exceed 95% in experienced centers to less than 60% in patients with unfavorable mitral valve anatomy.[20] A direct relationship exists between the experience of the interventional cardiologist performing the procedure and the incidence of procedural complications.[29] Most of the complications of the procedure including, mitral regurgitation, tamponade and a suboptimal improvement in mitral valve gradient are most often related to unfavorable mitral valve anatomy (represented by elevated Wilkin's scores).[7],[12] In contrast, patients with Wilkin's scores < 8 have a low rate of complications (< 2%), less re-stenosis and more than a 90% chance of procedure success.[20]

7. Mitral regurgitation

While mild mitral regurgitation is a common outcome following PBMV and is an understandable consequence of commissurotomy, acute severe mitral regurgitation is fortunately a rare complication that develops when the balloon commissurotomy produces a leaflet(s) tear, damages the sub-valvular compartment and/or causes chordae rupture. This may require emergent surgical correction.[19],[27] Severe mitral regurgitation is most often seen in patients with severe orifice narrowing, severely diseased leaflets and significant sub-valvular disease.[20]

The Brockenbrough procedure creates an iatrogenic inter-atrial septal defect, which usually carries no hemodynamic significance. However, hemo-pericardium can occur with perforation of adjacent structures by the Brockenbrough needle with an incidence of 2.0 %.[20] Manipulation of the catheter in the mitral valve position can lead to an unintended perforation of the left atrium, left atrial appendage, pulmonary veins, ventricular wall or apex, or aortic root. These complications can be readily avoided using real-time 3D echocardiography, which can promptly identify a pericardial effusion and help guide catheterization equipment in intracardiac structures.

8. Procedural guidance and assessment of results

Currently, real-time 3D trans-esophageal echocardiography (RT3DTEE) is often used in the catheterization laboratory to guide the various steps involved in performing a PBMV procedure,[30] (Figures 8 and 9) as the guide-wires, catheters and devices used during the procedure may not be readily apparent when using 2D trans-esophageal echocardiography. RT3DTEE,

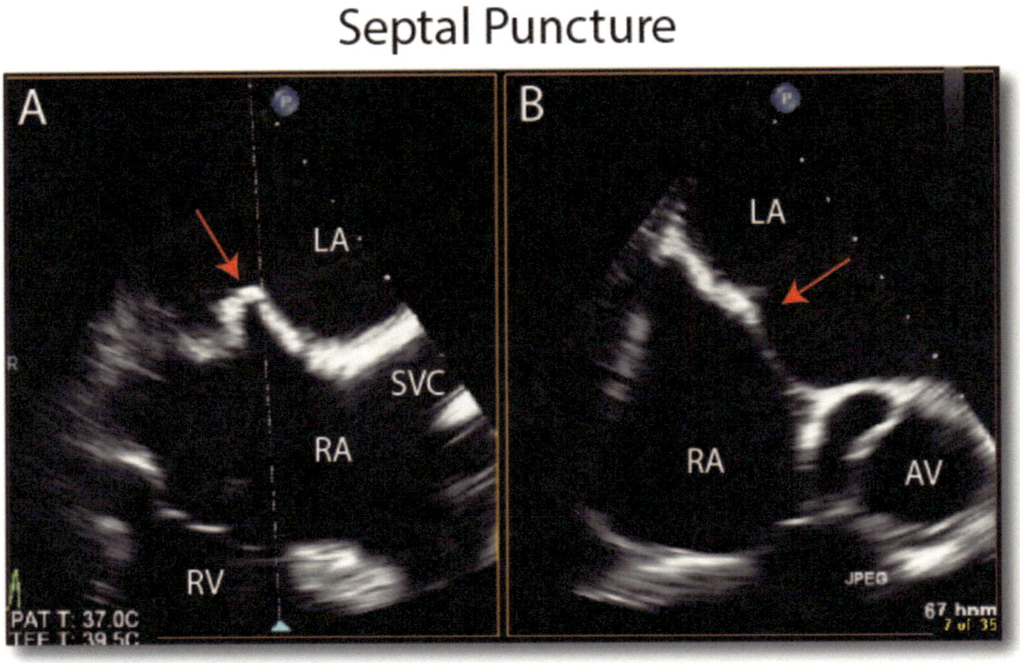

LA: left atrium; RA: right atrium; SVC: superior vena cava; AV: aortic valve

Figure 8. transeptal puncture is usually the first step in the mitral valve balloon valvuloplasty. Transesophageal echocardiography now plays a central role for guiding this procedure. Simultaneous biplane imaging is the preferred TEE guiding mode. Panel A depicts a bicaval view with the Brockenbrough needle tenting (red arrow) the interatrial septum at the level of the fossa ovalis. In panel B the same is illustrated from an orthogonal view at the level of the aortic valve.

particularly presented in the x plane format, can effectively visualize the precise location of the tenting of the septum during septal puncture, thereby increasing the safety of this critical step.[31] Moreover, real-time 3DTEE can more accurately assess MVA and mitral regurgitation before and after valvuloplasty, compared to 2DE. RT3DTEE allows for imaging the valve during balloon dilation, "en face" and possibly avoiding leaflet damage by stepwise balloon over-dilatation by visualizing commissural splitting and leaflet tears immediately after balloon dilation.[31] 3D TEE is also useful to help determine whether the balloon is free of the chordal stuctures prior to inflation. RT3DTEE can accurately determine when optimal MVA balloon dilatation has been achieved and the procedure can be successfully completed.

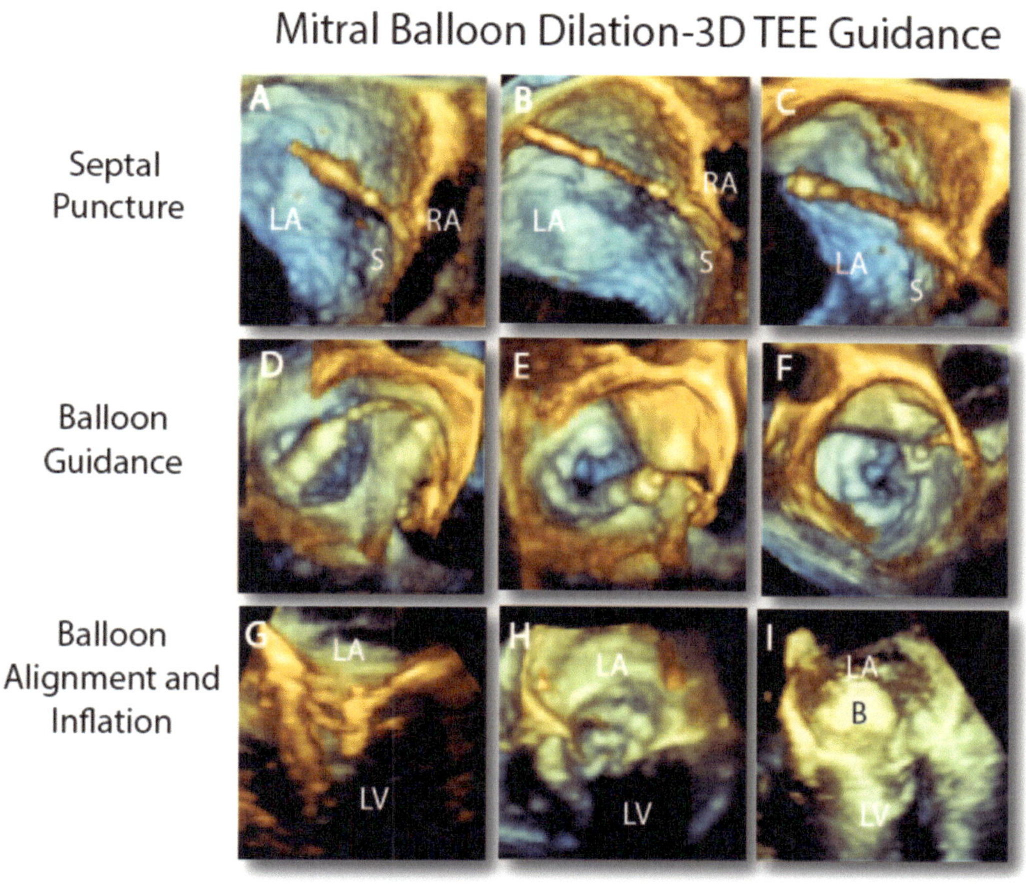

Figure 9. Three D TEE guidance is now commonly used to assist with all the phases of mitral balloon valvuloplasty. In panels A, B and C septal puncture is accomplished and the catheter is advanced through the inter-atrial septum (S) from the right atrium (RA) to the left atrium (LA). In panels D, E and F the balloon is guided to the mitral orifice and finally through the mitral valve into the left ventricle. In panels G and H the balloon is aligned to the long axis of the left ventricle (LV) and in panel I the balloon is inflated.

9. Conclusion

Percutaneous balloon mitral valvuloplasty has become the first line of treatment in individuals with symptomatic rheumatic mitral stenosis.

Echocardiographic imaging plays a pivotal role in both the diagnosis of mitral stenosis as well as the guidance of catheter-based procedures (e.g., PBMV) used in treatment. With the advancement of ultrasound imaging real-time 3D echocardiography supplements current 2D technology and offers an advantage over conventional echocardiography for the evaluation of patients being considered for percutaneous balloon mitral valvuloplasty. With the large number of factors that play a role in determining patients suitability for PBMV as well the risk for poor outcomes, further defining patient anatomy with advanced imaging such as real-time 3D echocardiography should improve both short and long-term outcomes.

Author details

Mark A. Navarro, Michael Kim and Ernesto E. Salcedo

*Address all correspondence to: ernesto.e.salcedo@ucdenver.edu

University of Colorado, Hospital Anschutz Medical Campus, USA

References

[1] Dean, L. S. Percutaneous transvenous mitral commissurotomy: a comparison to the closed and open surgical techniques. Cathet Cardiovasc Diagn.(1994). suppl 2):76-81.

[2] Baumgartner, H, Hung, J, Bermejo, J, et al. Echocardiographic assessment of valve stenosis: EAE/ASE recommendations for clinical practice. J Am Soc Echocardiogr. (2009). , 22, 1-23.

[3] Leopold, P, Casanova, C, Almeria, C, et al. Which method should be the reference method to evaluate the severity of rheumatic mitral stenosis? Gorlin's method versus 3D-echo. Eur J Echocardiography.(2007). , 8, 470-473.

[4] Thomas, J, Wilkins, G, Choong, C, et al. Inaccuracy of mitral pressure half-time immediately after percutaneous mitral valvotomy: dependence on transmitral gradient and left atrial and ventricular compliance. Circulation.(1988). , 78, 980-93.

[5] Perez de Isla LCasanova C, Almeria C, et al. Which method should be the reference method to evaluate the severity of rheumatic mitral stenosis? Gorlin's method versus 3D-echo.Eur J Echocardiography.(2007). , 8, 470-473.

[6] Zamorano, J. Perez de Isla L, Sugeng L et al. Non-invasive assessment of mitral valve area during percutaneous balloon mitral valvuloplasty: role of real-time 3D echocardiography. European heart journal (2004)., 25, 2086-91.

[7] Messika-zeitoun, D, Iung, B, Brochet, E, et al. Evaluation of mitral stenosis in (2008). Archives of Cardiovascular Disease.2008; , 101, 653-663.

[8] Binder, T. M, Risenhek, R, Porenta, G, Maurer, G, & Baumgartner, H. Improved Assessment of Mitral Valve Stenosis by Volumetric Real-Time Three-Dimensional Echocardiography. Jounral of the American College of Cardiology.(2000)., 36, 1355-61.

[9] Anwar, A. M, Attia, W. M, Nosir, Y. F, et al. Validation of a new score for the assessment of mitral stenosis using real-time three-dimensional echocardiography. Journal of the American Society of Echocardiography : official publication of the American Society of Echocardiography.(2010)., 23, 13-22.

[10] Messika-zeitoun, D, Brochet, E, Holmin, C, et al. Three-dimensional evaluation of the mitral valve area and commissural opening before and after percutaneous mitral commissurotomy in patients with mitral stenosis. European heart journal.(2007)., 28, 72-79.

[11] Dreyfus, J, Brochet, E, Lepage, L, et al. Real-time 3D transoesophageal measurement of the mitral valve area in patients with mitral stenosis. European journal of echocardiography : the journal of the Working Group on Echocardiography of the European Society of Cardiology (2011)., 12, 750-5.

[12] Wilkin, G. T, Weyman, A. E, Abascal, V. M, et al. Percutaneous balloon dilatation of the mitral valve: an analysis of echocardiographic variables realted to outcome and the mechanism of dilitation. Br Heart J. (1998)., 60, 299-308.

[13] Iung, B, Cormier, B, Ducimetiere, P, et al. Immediate results of percutaneous mitral commissurotomy. A predictive model on a series of 1514 patients. Circulation. (1996)., 94, 2124-2130.

[14] Padial, L. R, Freitas, N, Sagie, A, et al. Echocardiography can predict which patients will develop severe mitral regurgitation after percutaneous mitral balloon valvulotomy. J Am Coll Cardiol.(1996)., 27, 1225-1231.

[15] Cannan, C. R, Nishimura, R. A, Reeder, G. S, et al. Echocardiographic assessment of commissural calcium: a simple predictor of outcome after percutaneous mitral balloon valvotomy. J Am Coll Cardiol. (1997)., 29, 175-180.

[16] Sutaria, N, Northridge, D. B, & Shaw, T. R. Significance of commissural calcium on outcome of mitral balloon valvotomy. Heart.(2000)., 84, 398-402.

[17] Bonow, R. O, Carabello, B. A, Chatterjee, K, et al. ACC/AHA (2006). guidelines for the management of patients with valvular heart disease: a report of the American College of Cardiology/American Heart Association Task Force on Practice Guidelines. J Am Coll Cardiol.2006;48:ee148., 1.

[18] Iung, B, Garbarz, E, Michaud, P, et al. Late results of percutaneous mitral commissure in a series of 1024 patients. Circulation.(1999). , 99, 3272-3278.

[19] Iung, B, & Vahanian, A. The Long-term Outcome of Balloon Valvuloplasty for Mitral Stenosis. Current Cardiology Reports.(2002). , 4, 118-124.

[20] Nobuyoshi, M, Arita, T, Shirai, S, et al. Percutaneous balloon mitral valvuloplasty: a review. Circulation.(2009). e , 211-9.

[21] Hernandez, R, Banuelos, C, Alfonso, F, et al. Long-term clinical and echocardiographic follow-up after percutaneous mitral valvuloplasty with the Inoue balloon. Circulation. (1999). , 99, 1580-1586.

[22] Chmielak, Z, Klopotowski, M, Kruk, M, et al. Repeat percutaneous mitral balloon valvuloplasty for patients with mitral valve restenosis. Cathet. Cardiovasc. Intervent. (2010).

[23] Song, J. K, Song, J. M, Kang, D. M, et al. Restenosis and adverse clinical events after unsuccessful percutaneous mitral valvuloplasty: immediate post-procedural mitral valve area as an important prognostic factor. Eur Heart J. (2009). , 30, 1254-1262.

[24] Fawzy, M. E, Shoukri, H. K, Al-buraki, J, et al. Seventeen years' clinical and echocardiographic follow up of mitral balloon valvuloplasty in 520 patients and predictors of long-term outcome. J Heart Valve Dis.(2007). , 16, 454-460.

[25] Ben-farhat, M, Betbout, F, Gamra, H, et al. Predictors of long-term event free survival and freedom from restenosis after percutaneous balloon mitral commissurotomy. AM Heart J. (2001). , 142, 1072-1079.

[26] Palacios, I. F, Sanchez, P. L, Harrell, L. C, et al. Which patients benefit from percutaneous mitral balloon valvuloplasty? Prevalvuloplasty and postvalvuloplasty variables that predict long-term outcome. Circulation.(2002). , 105, 1465-1471.

[27] Cohen, D, Kuntz, R, Gordon, S, et al. Predictors of Long-term Outcome After Percutaneous Balloon Mitral Valvuloplasty. N Engl J Med. (1992). , 327, 1329-1335.

[28] Fawzy, M. E. Long-Term Results up to 19 Years of Mitral Balloon Valvuloplasty. Asian Cardiovascular & Thoracic Annals.(2009). , 17, 627-633.

[29] Complications and mortality of percutaneous mitral balloon commissurotomyA report from the National Heart, Lung and Blood Institute Balloon Valvuloplasty Registry. Circulation.(1992). , 85, 2014-2024.

[30] Eng, M. H, Salcedo, E. E, Quaife, R, et al. Implementation of Real Time Three-Dimensional Transesophageal Echocardiography in Percutaneous Mitral Balloon Valvuloplasty and Structural Heart Disease Interventions. Echocardiography.(2009). , 26, 958-966.

http://dx.doi.org/10.5772/56433

[31] Applebaum, R. M, Ksaliwal, R. R, Kanojia, A, et al. Utility of three-dimensional echocardiography during balloon mitral valvuloplasty. J Am Coll Cardiol. (1998). , 32, 1405-1409.

Chapter 6

A Framework for the Systematic Characterization of the Aortic Valve Complex by Real-Time Three Dimensional Echocardiography: Implications for Transcatheter Aortic Valve Replacement

Daniel Zalkind, Michael Kim and Ernesto E. Salcedo

Additional information is available at the end of the chapter

http://dx.doi.org/10.5772/56021

1. Introduction

Transcatheter aortic valve replacement (TAVR) has become a viable alternative to surgical aortic valve replacement in both high-risk and inoperable patients with symptomatic severe aortic stenosis [1]. A successful TAVR procedure is heavily dependent on appropriate patient selection and detailed morphologic characterization of the aortic valve complex to prevent device migration, coronary artery compromise and paravalvular leak. Two-dimensional echocardiography (2DE) and Doppler methods have traditionally been used to characterize the presence and severity of aortic stenosis [2]; however the detailed structural analysis of the aortic valve complex required for successful TAVR demands a more precise analysis of not only the aortic leaflets, but of the left ventricular outflow tract dimensions, aortic valve annulus, and the aortic root. Computed tomography (CT) [3, 4, 5, 6] and two dimensional transesophageal echocardiography (2D TEE) [7] are traditionally used to obtain this information. Although transthoracic and transesophageal three-dimensional echocardiography (3D Echo) provide detailed characterization of the aortic valve complex, these advanced modalities are not currently being routinely used in the evaluation of patients considered for TAVR. The purpose of this chapter is to provide a framework for the 3D echocardiographic evaluation of the aortic valve complex and its implications for TAVR.

1.1. The aortic valve complex

The aortic valve complex includes the aortic valve leaflets and surrounding structures defining a functional unit that allows, under normal circumstances, unidirectional and unobstructed blood flow to exit the left ventricle and to enter the ascending aorta. The clinical anatomy of the aortic root has been well characterized in other publications [8, 9] and is summarized below. More recently, the anatomy of the aortic valve complex and its implications in TAVR have been elegantly reviewed by Piazza [10]. The components of the aortic valve complex are illustrated in (Figure 1).

2. Anatomy and clinical application

2.1. General anatomical landmarks

As described above, the aortic annulus is one part of the aortic valve complex that is comprised of the muscular ventricular LVOT, the aortic valve, aortic leaflets, sinuses of Valsalva, the sinotubular junction and the ascending aorta [11]. The aortic annulus diameter and general geometry, which is crucial for pre-procedural planning, valve implantation and post-procedural follow-up can be considered to be a virtual ring joining the basal attachments of all three aortic valve cusps, representing the inlet from the left ventricular outflow tract into the aortic root [12]. The annulus described by surgeons is usually the semilunar crown-like structure demarcated by the hinges of the leaflets. There is also the true ring, comprised of the sinotubular junction, demarcated by the sinus ridge and the related sites of attachment of the peripheral zones of apposition between the aortic valve leaflets. This forms the outlet of the aortic root into the ascending aorta.

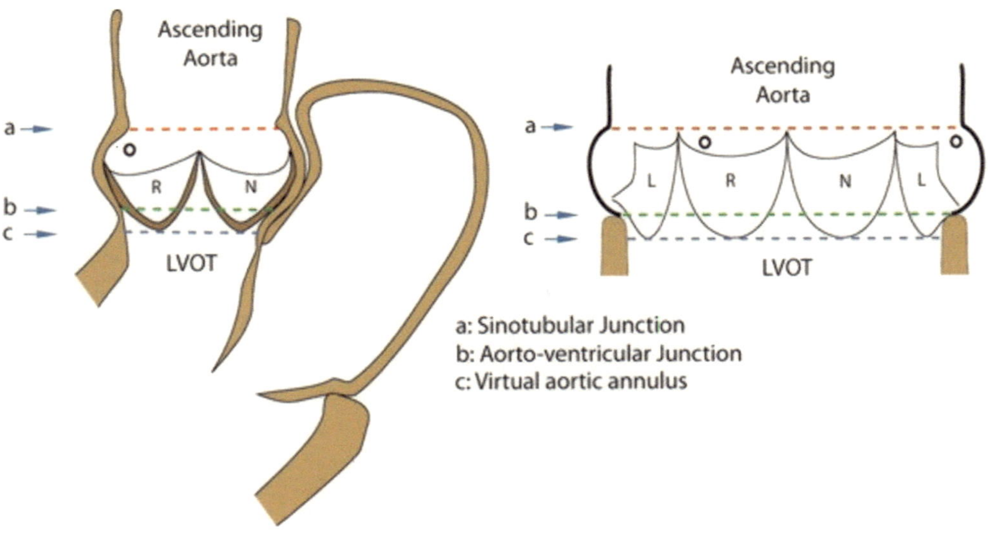

Figure 1. Aortic valve complex with virtual and anatomical rings.

The larger part of the noncoronary leaflet of the valve, along with part of the left coronary leaflet, is in fibrous continuity with the aortic or anterior leaflet of the mitral valve,

http://dx.doi.org/10.5772/56021

with the ends of this area of fibrous continuity being thickened to form the so-called fibrous trigones. It is these trigones that anchor the aortic-mitral valvular unit to the roof of the left ventricle. The valvular complex is a dynamic structure, with the geometric parameters changing continuously during the phases of the cardiac cycle and in relation to changes in pressure within the aortic root. From diastole to systole, the change in the diameter at the level of the outlet and at the base of the valve has been noted to increase more than 10%, according to several earlier publications. Proper functioning of the native aortic valve depends on the proper relationship between the leaflets within the aortic root. Not only do variations exist among individuals in the dimensions of the root, but in the same individual, marked variations can exist in all aspects of the dimensions of the individual leaflets, including the height, width, surface area, and volume of each of the supporting sinuses of Valsalva.

2.2. Application of echocardiography

Transthoracic echocardiography (TTE) is a critical portion of patient selection for TAVR and complements the clinical criteria for TAVR due to its robust ability to provide both anatomical and hemodynamic data. According to the latest European Association of Echocardiography and the ASE 2011 consensus document [13], the role of TTE is to specifically assess the annular dimension and detailed anatomic characteristics of the aortic valve, including the number, mobility, and thickness of cusps, as well as the extent and distribution of calcification.

Patients being considered for TAVR should undergo a pre-TAVR 2D/Doppler TTE evaluation to serve as a baseline for post-TAVR comparison. In addition 3D TTE should be performed to more precisely delineate the aortic valve complex in order to better determine patient suitability for TAVR. Transthoracic echo plays a key role in establishing the presence of severe AS with Doppler assessment of peak and mean transaortic gradients as well as AVA calculation by the continuity equation. Per the current ACC/AHA guidelines, severe AS is defined by an AVA of <1cm2 (<0.6 cm2/m2) or a mean aortic valve gradient of >40 mmHg. The aortic valvular dimension must be assessed with echocardiography, as the current guidelines recommend a 23 mm prosthesis for transverse aortic annular diameters of 18–21 mm (measured at the level of aortic cusp insertion) and a 26 mm prosthesis for aortic annular diameters of 22–25 mm. There is also a larger 29mm SAPIEN valve which is currently available outside of the United States which can accommodate 26-29mm annular diameters.

Using TTE, assessing the annular dimension and detailed anatomic characteristics of the aortic valve, including the number, mobility, and thickness of cusps, as well as the extent and distribution of calcification should be described. LV and right ventricular dimensions and function, aortic regurgitation, and the structure and function of the other valves should be evaluated. Other valvular disease such as severity of valvular regurgitation or presence of bioprothetic valves in other positions must also be closely evaluated as such findings may preclude TAVR. Left ventricular thrombus and valvular vegetations must be ruled out due to the risk of embolization during sheath manipulation prior to or during deployment. LVOT obstruction and calcification should also be evaluated as it can interfere with device deployment and can lead to migration of the valve. Pericardial fibrosis or pericardial patch should be evaluated with either echocardiography or CT as the transapical approach requires a thoracotomy and pericardioctemy.

During the implantation of a transcatheter aortic valve, contact between the valve struts or between the mechanically dilated and moved native calcifications can skirt the membranous septum, potentially instigating high-degree atrioventricular heart block caused by the compression of the left bundle. This phenomenon is of particular concern in patients with pre-existing right bundle branch block (RBBB).

Currently, bicuspid aortic valve is an exclusion criterion for TAVR because an elliptical valvular orifice may predispose to an increased risk of incomplete and incorrect deployment of the aortic prosthesis, predisposing to a risk of paravalvular leak or valve embolization post implantation. Moreover, the risk of aortic complications in patients with bicuspid aortic valves, such as spontaneous aortic dissection, may be increased due to abnormal arterial wall structure.

2.3. Aortic and mitral valve interaction

Although difficult to study and to characterize with traditional 2D echocardiography, the interaction between the mitral and aortic valves can vary in intensity and may have subtle effects on the success or failure of TAVR. A study of this interaction from Veronesi and colleagues demonstrated that the interaction between the mitral annulus surface area and aortic annulus projected area changed reciprocally over time due to the physical interaction through this fibrous continuity [14]. The aortic annulus projected area increased 17% from end diastole to early systole and decreased to a minimum during isovolumic relaxation. The angle between the mitral and aortic annuli decreased by 5% from diastole to systole. It is reasonable to infer that valve undersizing, resulting in more frequent and/or severe perivalvular aortic regurgitation, may result if the coupling between the aortic and mitral valves is not appreciated. Other work in mitral-aortic valve coupling was presented at the ACC conference in 2012 and described that aortic stenosis patients have reduced mitral annular size and displacement. After TAVR, mitral annular size remains reduced due to the presence of the calcified aortic valve, which is compressed along the aortic root by the TAVR valve struts. This may also contribute to the increase in aortic-mitral angle post-TAVI [15].

2.4. General Description of the Sinuses of Valsalva and coronary artery ostia

The aortic root is a geometrically complicated structure that includes the sinuses of Valsalva which are in direct communication with the coronary cusp insertion points. The coronary artery ostia are in the sinuses and thus give name to the sinuses (left, right and non-coronary) [16]. The height of the sinuses and the proximity to the aortic valve cusps in systole are two important parameters to consider in the pre-TAVR planning

For pre-TAVR planning, the LVOT view (110-140 degrees of omni-plane) should be used to visualize the height of the sinus, defined as the distance from the aortic annulus to the sinotubular junction (tapering of the sinuses to the ascending aorta diameter) [17]. We have found success in visualizing the sinuses of Valsalva with transthoracic 3D by using multi-plane reconstruction (MPR) [18] and measuring the longest diameter and area. MPR can also be used to assess the height of the sinuses, best visualized with our technique from the "Full Volume" acquisition from the parasternal long window as shown in figures 2-4. Alternatively, CT imaging can also be used with a similar MPR technique.

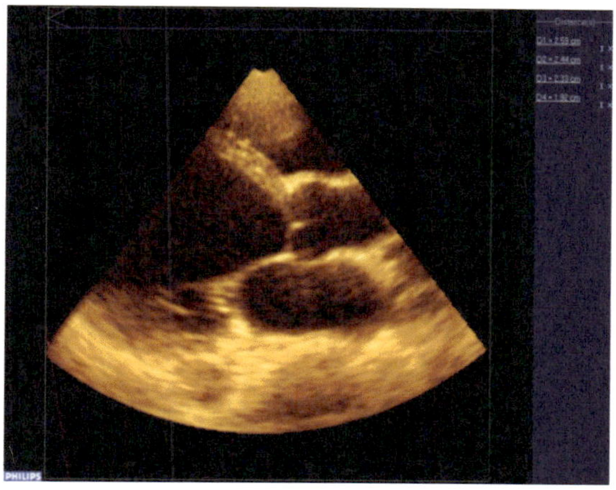

Figure 2. LVOT view from parasternal long MPR

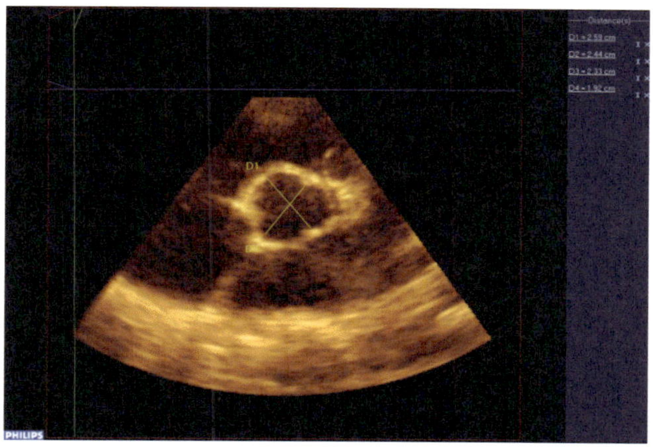

Figure 3. Aortic annular dimension from parasternal long MPR

2.5. Fibrous interleaflet triangles

The portion of the aortic wall that is beneath the apices formed by the attachment of the aortic leaflets straddles the ventricular and aortic sides of the aortic valve. This region of the heart is exposed to the ventricular hemodynamic forces. Also known as trigones, these structures help to support the integrity of the aortic valve [19]. Some authors have made the analogy to a suspension bridge where the collagenous thickening at the zone of coaptation and the hinges

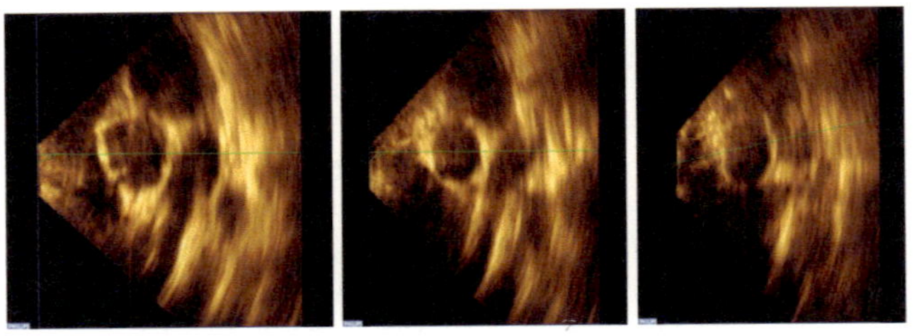

Figure 4. Sinus of valsva (left), sinotubular junction (center) and ascending aorta (right). MPR from parasternal long view.

of the leaflets correspond to support cables. These interleaflet triangles are crucial for proper valvular function. When one or more of them are vestigial, or very small, the valve can become stenotic due to a change in the geometry. It is challenging to view these structures with transthoracic echocardiography but TEE can sometime be used to identify them if the valvular motion is slowed down during the post-processing stage and they are identified in mid systole or possibly mid diastole, depending on the plane of imaging that is used. Three-dimensional echocardiography does not quite have the resolution to discriminate between these thin structures and the valve leaflets. These triangles are currently not part of the TAVR planning protocols at most institutions at this time.

2.6. Tubular portion of ascending aorta

Aortic valvular disease such as aortic stenosis and aortic regurgitation can often be accompanied by ascending aortic dilatation. In a recent, large case series from Baylor Medical Center, of the 1385 patients who had isolated aortic valve replacement, 59 also had aortic root resection [20]. The largest ascending aortic diameter (multiple imaging modalities were included) ranged from 4.5 to 6.7 cm (mean, 5.3+-0.5 cm): these diameters were larger in the men than in the women (mean, 5.4 cm versus mean, 4.9 cm). Although the association between bicuspid valve and aortopathy is well known, occasionally patient with severe AS may be referred for TAVR and the valve is so heavily calcified that the diagnosis of bicuspid valve (and thus their ineligibility for TAVR) is not known. Wide-sector acquisition in the left parasternal long axis can be used to visualize the ascending aorta and thus help to identify dilatation of the ascending aorta that may, in itself, warrant surgical correction. Alternatively, CT with contrast can be used to assess the ascending aorta.

2.7. Aorto-mitral fibrosa

The aorto-mitral fibrosa is usually a thin piece of fibrous tissue that lies between the mitral and aortic annuli. Best visualized in the parasternal long view on TTE, the fibrosa is usually thin [21]. Alternations to the geometry of the left ventricular inflow and outflow regions can lead to variations in the length of this fibrosa, such as in transposition of the great vessels, endocarditis or heavy calcification of either or both annuli. From parasternal short axis window, acquisition can be performed in "Live 3D Zoom" modality to examine the left ventricular outflow tract and mitral valve region. More detailed pictures can, of course, be obtained with TEE as well.

http://dx.doi.org/10.5772/56021

2.8. Pathology including subvalvular stenosis and HCM

Echocardiography has been used to assess all of the structures mentioned above as well as hypertrophic cardiomyopathy (HCM) with substantial validation. In a thorough study of 77 pediatric patients with subaortic stenosis from the University of Michigan from 1983 to 1991, echocardiography was used to evaluate patients before and after surgical repair as well as follow them longitudinally as their gradients increased. In the 36 patients who underwent surgery, the pre-operative LVOT gradient decreased from 63 to 14mmHg [22]. TTE examinations were crucial in this patient population due to the complexity of the lesions. A discrete fibrous membrane or fibromuscular collar can frequently encircle the LVOT just beneath the aortic valve. Occasionally the long fibromuscular obstruction narrows the LVOT for several centimeters forming a tunnel. Accompanying aortic regurgitation can also be present and has been used as an indicator for urgent surgical correction. Three dimensional echocardiography can be especially useful in such cases as the aortic valvular pathology can be differentiated from the subaortic pathology and the aortic regurgitation can be fully described (eccentricity, vena contracta width and PISA) using 2D, 3D, pulsed doppler and color-flow doppler. Subaortic stenosis is a contraindication to CoreValve implantation. Additionally, the high incidence of concominant atrial and ventricular septal defects increases the utility of echocardiography as those defects can be readily visualized.

Hypertrophic cardiomyopathy (HCM) is the most common genetic cardiomyopathy with a prevalence of approximately 0.2%. The clinical presentation is quite diverse but the sentinel findings of either concentric basal hypertrophy (with septal involvement), arrhythmias and sudden cardiac death can be recognized late in the disease process [23]. According to the 2011 American Society of Echocardiography guidelines for HCM, ventricular volumes, discrete wall thickness and LV geometry (apical vs. septal hypertrophy) can be defined. Dynamic obstruction of the LVOT during stress can be assessed but due to the need for continuous wave Doppler, can be confused with severe aortic stenosis. In the evaluation of patients with suspected concominant aortic stenosis and a dynamic LVOT obstruction from HCM, TEE imaging is crucial to separate the two pathologies. Additionally, papillary muscle hypertrophy/remodeling can also lead to the elongation of the mitral leaflet area and lead to further increases in the LVOT gradient due to the venture effect in the hypertrophied and/or hyperdynamic LVOT. These dynamic processes must be evaluated prior to any consideration of transcatheter treatment of aortic stenosis.

3. Three dimensional echocardiography of the aortic valve complex

3.1. Background, physics and validation

Two dimensional echocardiography has numerous limitations in assessing the volumes and geometry of complex cardiac structures such as the left ventricular cavity (for the purposes of LVEF assessment) as described above and include geometric assumptions, image plane positioning errors and imprecise endocardial boundary demarcation [24]. Over the last twenty years, numerous advances in ultrasound transducer technology and parallel computer processing has made the acquisition of 3D echocardiographic volumes possible using multiple formats (in the Philips Healthcare system but similar modes in the other manufacturers as well) including large sector ("Full Volume"), narrow sector format ("Live 3D"), wide sector focused ("Zoom 3D"), simultaneous biplane ("X-plane") modes. The different formats are provided because 3D echocardiography is a technically demanding technique with temporal and spatial resolution limitations. Each one of the formats or modes has strengths and weaknesses.

One of the first clinical studies documenting real-time 3D echocardiography was published in 1998. The phased-array volumetric 3D system was developed in the Duke University Center for Emerging Cardiovascular Technology and initially operated with 2.5- or 3.4-MHz transducers (both 14 mm in diameter) [25]. A 2D array and the pyramid-shaped volumetric scan composed of 43x 43 square elements, each measuring 0.3x0.3 mm. The volume was scanned rapidly with 16-to-1 parallel processing in the receive system. Consequently, the overall scanned pyramidal volume was composed

of 256 small pyramids stacked side by side. Since then the transducer technology has increased substantially and current systems are solid state devices that operate at 5-7 MHz and are composed of more than 3000 array elements with the ability to acquire in the multiple modes above as well as to perform other advanced functions such as 3D color Doppler and color M-mode. This technology has been validated against nuclear magnetic resonance [26] and SPECT imaging [27].

Large sector acquisition ("Full Volume" on the Philips Healthcare system) is a technique for acquiring large volume sets such as the entire left ventricle over multiple cardiac cycles to allow the transducer/processor to sample small sectors of the entire volume during each cycle. The sectors are then "stitched" together by software algorithms into one large volume. This technique allows for large volumes to be imaged but relies on a regular heart rhythm that produces constant R-R intervals. Respiratory artifact can also be introduced if the ultrasound probe is affected leading to slightly different cardiac geometry to be sampled in the various sectors leading to "stitch" artifact. This technique has been used in our laboratory to define LV geometry as well to define the aortic annulus and the entirety of the aortic valve complex and proximal ascending aorta in one acquisition step. Apical and parasternal long positions are favored for this approach.

Narrow sector format ("Live 3D") is a technique which focuses on a narrow sector such as the aortic leaflets at the level of the Sinuses of Valsalva with high temporal resolution and frame rates above 30Hz for visualization of rapidly moving structures such as fenestrations, vegetations or thrombi. Temporal resolution is now sufficient to visualize valvular motion as seen in figure 5.

Wide sector focused ("Zoom 3D") allows for large acquisition fields that are relatively shallow which can be obtained anywhere along the long axis of the field of view. For example, the entire aortic valve annulus, leaflets and possibly the coronary ostia can be visualized. This approach is often coupled with the simultaneous orthogonal view format known as "X-plane". This 2D technique allows the sonographer to visualize complex structures in their traditional

http://dx.doi.org/10.5772/56021

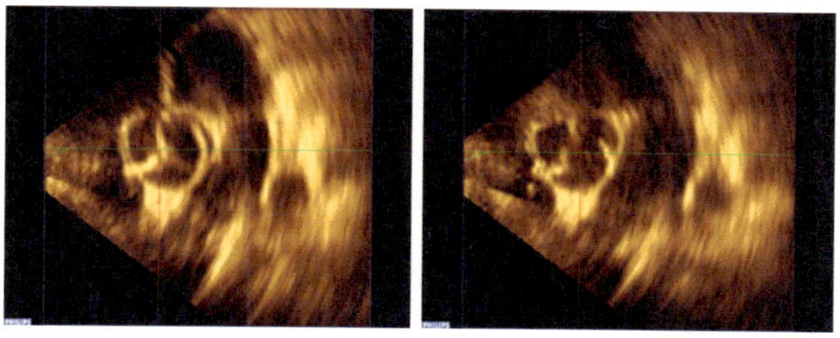

Figure 5. Aortic valve in diastole and systole with transthoracic 3D MPR reconstruction.

2D view and concurrently, in a split window format, visualize the orthogonal 2D plane. Especially useful in the identification of the coronary ostia and left atrial appendage thrombi and the aortic annular diameter.

3.2. Role for 3D echo from EAE and ASE guidelines

Since the development of the matrix-array transducer and real-time 3D echocardiography, the application to clinical practice has increased substantially due to improves accuracy and ease of use. Direct measurements of cardiac chambers without geometrical assumptions, non-invasive views of valvular structure and function as well as color Doppler assessment of regurgitation and stenosis are all improving and are gradually becoming well accepted and strongly recommended in the ASE guidelines [28].

Specifically 3D LV chamber quantification is now recommended as the best technique for evaluating LV end-diastolic and end-systolic volumes, leading to accurate quantification of LV ejection fraction. Several studies have now directly compared the accuracy of 3D measurements of LV volumes and EF have shown the superiority of the 3D approach over the 2D methodology, which was shown to consistently underestimate LV volumes.

Valvular heart disease has been studied as a possible application for RT3D as well. The most experience comes in mitral disease where the hyperbolic paraboloid ("saddle-shaped") geometry of the valve is better evaluated from multiple planes that are possible with 3D imaging. The current TAVR recommendations recommend that the aortic valve is imaged with 3D but the sizing of the valve still be performed with 2D echo in the LVOT view, usually accomplished at the mid-esophageal position at 120 degrees of omni tilt. LVOT measurements performed on the 3D dataset require multi-planar reconstruction (see below).

3.3. Wide-sector acquisition and advances in post processing

Although not currently endorsed for the pre-procedural evaluation for TAVR, transthoracic 3D imaging may have a special niche. Similar 3D capabilities as transesophageal echocardiography are available to the sonographer including RT3D with high-frame rate imaging (Live 3D) as well as breath-hold, large sector acquisition. The off-line processing software is currently aimed for LV ejection fraction quantification but, in the authors' experience, can be applied to the LVOT, aortic annulus and possibly the ascending aorta.

Three-dimensional imaging requires optimal patient positioning to minimize the lung space between the thoracic wall and the myocardium (extreme left decubitus) along with minimal subcutaneous fat layer. For example we typically perform apical 3D imaging on dedicated echocardiography tables with fold-out windows to allow for proper transducer alignment with the long-axis of the LV. This is crucial for 3D imaging of the LVOT [29] as the focus is more on the imaginary line drawn through the proximal ascending aorta into the LV cavity as we have found that the acquisition volume needs to be positioned over the aortic valvular complex and the ascending aorta.

Often the increased calcium in the aortic annulus and on the leaflets causes shadowing of the aortic valve and ascending aorta. We have found that parasternal long 3D imaging with both Live3D and Full-Volume acquisition produces easily interpretable and physiologic images [30]. This view is crucial for highly calcified aortic valves or for HCM patient with substantially hypertrophied septum which can be calcified and can obstruct the aortic annulus.

Once the 3D sample volume is acquired in either the "Full Volume" or "Zoom 3D" formats, multi-plane reconstruction can be used to visualize the aortic valve complex in any plane. Most useful for the assessment of the aortic annular diameter as well as the diameter of the sino-tubular junction, MPR allows the echocardiographer to solve the issue of "oblique" planes through round structures that can lead to under or overestimation of the annular diameter. In a recent retrospective analysis in the Journal of the American College of Cardiology, Wilson and colleagues suggested that CT imaging of the aortic annulus is more accurate and can lead to better sizing for TAVR, presumably leading to less perivalvular regurgitation (See below for the unique benefits of 3D echocardiography in perivalvular regurgitation).

An off-line processing feature on the Philips workstation known as "I-Slice" is an automatic software feature that isolates multiple segments of the LV and allows for separate evaluation. Mostly designed for the evaluation of LV function throughout different segments of the chamber, this feature can also be applied to the transthoracic evaluation of the aortic valve complex and the ascending aorta by applying it along the LVOT-to-ascending aorta axis. Orthogonal 2D slices at multiple levels of this area of interest can be displayed simultaneously and thus can help to identify calcium, maximal and minimal diameters and areas of supra-aortic and sub-aortic stenosis without the need for multi-plane reconstruction (Fig. 6).

4. Clinical application in aortic stenosis

The publication of the PARTNER trial ushered in a new era in interventional cardiology and highlights the improved outcomes of TAVR vs. medical treatment. As originally reported by Braunwald and colleagues and recently further explored by Carabello and colleagues, aortic stenosis had a 2% incidence in the Cardiovascular Health Study and has a high mortality rate (especially with symptoms) when medical treatment alone is initiated. As per the 2008 EAE/ASE valvular guidelines, echocardiography has become the standard means for evaluation of aortic stenosis (AS) severity [31]. Cardiac catheterization

http://dx.doi.org/10.5772/56021

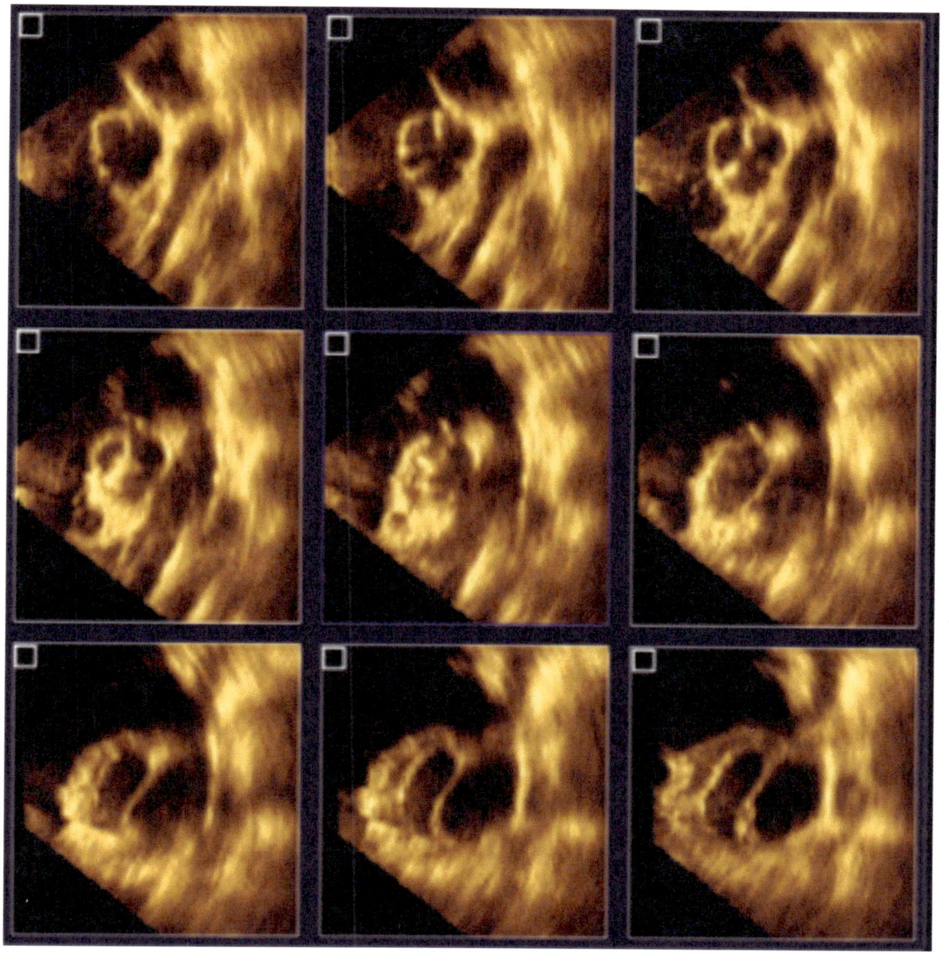

Figure 6. Philips "I-Slice" mode applied to the aortic valve complex.

is no longer recommended except in rare cases when echocardiography is non-diagnostic or discrepant with clinical data [32].

As mentioned above, non-invasive imaging including echocardiography is important and plays a central role in TAVR because accurate preoperative measurements of aortic annular sizes are crucial for selection of appropriate prosthesis sizes. One of the possible imaging modalities, 2D echocardiography underestimates aortic annular and LVOT dimensions compared when compared with multislice computed tomography (MSCT) and 3D echocardiography [33]. Three dimensional TEE has been promoted for more accurate diameter measurements. A study by Ng and colleagues, from the Netherlands, showed marked differences in the aortic annular dimension measurement between 2D TEE, 3D TEE circular annular assumption and 3D TEE with planimetry measurements based on overall valve area although all of the modalities were consistent when eccentricity was measured post TAVR (circular valve prosthesis). Using CT planimetered areas as "gold standard," 3D TEE planimetered aortic annular and LVOT areas showed the least underestimation and narrowest limits of agreements compared with their respective calculated circular areas. After TAVR, both 3D TEE and CT demonstrated a decrease in the annular dimension and area due to the thickness of the valve stent thickness [34]. In contrast, the planimetered LVOT areas increased by both modalities due to a more circular geometry after TAVR.

Three dimensional TEE has another niche in aortic stenosis. Obstructions in the LVOT or post-procedural complications such as pannus formation in surgical valves can be visualized with real time 3D TEE [35]. A pannus that formed on a mitral valve that could be visualized only with 3D TEE was reported by Ozkan and colleagues in 2009. The same technology technique could be transferred to the aortic valve with the caveat that shadowing can often complicate visualization of intra-valvular pathology, based on our experience.

Finally, two dimensional echocardiography has recently been used to estimate effective orifice area after TAVR and the measurement of the LVOT diameter immediately proximal to the valve stent struts produced the most likely true effective orifice area with the minimal false negative prosthesis-patient-mismatch (AVA <0.65cm/m2) [36].

4.1. Aortic insufficiency and perivalvular leaks

Periprocedural complications of device deployment may limit the short-term and long-term results that have been reported. One common problem is perivalvular aortic regurgitation. Two dimensional [37, 38] and three dimensional echo has been validated in native valve regurgitation in previous studies [39, 40, 41]. Based on the previous experience in surgically-implanted valves, periprosthetic leak severity is defined as severe when greater than 25% of the ring circumference is involved by color Doppler [42]. While predictors for left ventricular functional recovery or survival following valve replacement have been investigated, predictors for paravalvular aortic regurgitations after TAVR are less established. Postprocedural aortic regurgitation grade 2/4 has been noted in about 12–20% of patients. In a recent study by Koos and colleagues [43], pre-TAVR CT scans were performed to calculate the Agastson calcium score and the routine echocardiographical protocol was used for pre and post-TAVR [44]. There was a correlation between very high Agastson scores (over 3000) and aortic insufficiency ¾ and higher. In a recent retrospective study, Sherif and colleagues [45] performed a univariate regression analysis on 50 successful CoreValve deployments and found that the LVOT-Ao angle, oval LVOT shape and prior AI all contributed significantly to the development of ¾ or 4/4 aortic insufficiency. Three dimensional TEE is helpful in these cases as the geometry of the LV and the acuity of the differences in the LV axis and the LVOT-Ao axis, the shape of the LVOT and the amount of AI can all be assessed with 2D and 3D echocardiography. In a recent review of PARTNER I 2-year follow-up data, perivalvular regurgitation has been associated with increased mortality (Hazard ratio 2.11 for mild to moderate in severity). [46]

4.2. Echocardiography during deployment [47, 48, 49, 50, 51, 52]

The imaging modalities that have described previously in this text for the pre-procedural evaluation of the aortic valve complex have been compared to the Hegar dilator technique in the

http://dx.doi.org/10.5772/56021

work of Dashkevich and colleagues. Two dimensional TEE often underestimates the size of the aortic annulus when compared to CT that correlated well to the anatomical measurement. Whichever technique is used for sizing, the utility of live two and three dimensional echocardiography during the procedure is well accepted and outlined by Lerakis and colleagues.

The first step in the deployment of the Edwards-Sapien valve is achieving coaxiality of the delivery catheter with the LVOT-Aorta. This is best accomplished in the TEE probe in the high esophageal position, LVOT view, at 110-140 degrees of omniposition. Other authors have also recommended 3D TEE imaging with the use of "Zoom 3D" mode at 135, which allows a more precise positioning of the tip of the catheter and the prosthesis in relation to the aortic Annulus [53].

The next step is to align the aortic end of the THV with the tips of the native aortic valve leaflets. Fluoroscopy is used simultaneously and is discussed elsewhere [54]. After deployment, the 3-dimensional transesophageal echocardiography short-axis view of the THV can be used to show a successful outcome with normal valve function and color Doppler can be used to assess possible valvular or perivalvular regurgitation. Mild to moderate perivalvular regurgitation is common after TAVR with the CoreValve. Sizing based on mean annulus diameter may help to reduce according to one recent retrospective review of 50 patients [55].

In clinical practice, optimal positioning of the CoreValve 5-10mm proximal to the native aortic annulus occurs only 50% of the time by fluoroscopy. Non-optimal positioning has been found to have an inverse relationship to patient-prosthesis mismatch [56]. In our experience, the utility of TEE during deployment is greatest for recapturable valves such as the CoreValve as live evidence of perivalvular regurgitation can be useful before repositioning is performed. For Edwards-Sapien valves this is less crucial as the valve is deployed and cannot be recaptured. In very rare circumstances, the THV is deployed with the wrong orientation, thus producing severe, open valvular regurgitation. This can be assessed quickly with either 2D or 3D echo. Another valve is subsequently deployed within the inproperly deployed valve.

Positioning of the valve is critical as is the surveillance of the aortic valve complex and ascending aorta for any atheromas or loose calcium that can contribute to cerebrovascular accidents. There is no currently well-accepted description of the etiology of peri-procedural CVA.

Patient follow-up at three days post-procedure as well as months out is routine at our center. As with surgical aortic valve replacement, TTE is the imaging modality of choice for evaluation of prosthesis function during follow-up. Post-implantation gradients should be followed. There is flow acceleration at the valve stent as well as in the bioprosthetic valvular insertion point in the stent. This can lead to an overestimation of the trans-valvular gradients if the sample volume is placed inside the stent in the "subvalvular" position. As described above, the most proximal point of the stent should be used as the LVOT diameter and the sample volume should be placed there in the Doppler interrogation of the Edwards-Sapien valves [57]. Left ventricular hypertrophy should also be assessed. In fact, left ventricular hypertrophy that has been well described to be associated with clinically important aortic stenosis can be followed with transthoracic echocardiography and the Devereux formula in combination with the relative wall thickness has been used to evaluate the regression of increased ventricular wall thickness.

4.3. Limitations and alternative approaches

4.3.1. Cardiac computed tomography [58, 59, 60]

As with other cardiac structures, the cardiologist and cardiac surgeon has multiple imaging modalities available for the evaluation of the aortic valve complex for TAVR planning. As described by Bloomfield and colleagues in a recent review paper, multi-detector CT, cardiac MRI and, of course, fluoroscopy can all be used to assess the area of interest. There are numerous advantages and disadvantages to each technique [61]. Fluoroscopy and CT are discussed elsewhere in this chapter. Although cardiac CT can provide a MFR image for multiple measurements, the most reproducible MDCT measurements of the annulus are the area-derived diameter and basal ring average diameter, with derived values generally larger than those obtained with echocardiography. More recently, the annular circumference has begun to emerge as the gold standard [62].

4.3.2. Cardiac magnetic resonance imaging [63, 64]

Cardiac magnetic resonance allows for an anatomic and functional assessment of the aortic valve and aortic root. However, most CMR sequences are two-dimensional with the plane of imaging chosen at the time of the examination. Whole heart, echo-gated 3D cardiac MR can provide isotropic images for multiplanar reconstruction and shows the oval shape of the annulus with maximal and minimal diameters. Planimetric calculations can be made using steady-state free precession cine sequences. Limitations due to Gadollium contrast and long acquisition times are two reasons why it is less desirable and not routinely used in clinical practice.

5. Future directions

5.1. Single cardiac cycle imaging [65]

Although current limitations of 3D echo includes frame rate, acquisition volume and resolution there are both hardware and software advances coming in the future. Improvements in transducer design, parallel-processing and automated edge-detection and LV volume calculations will enable the sonographer to acquire higher quality images and the physician to answer clinical questions faster. Off-line processing will become simpler and less time consuming as well. Additional advances in the miniaturization of the probe and the echocardiogram machine itself will allow for wider use in the clinical setting.

6. Conclusions

Three dimensional echocardiography has emerged as a crucial imaging modality for TAVR planning and followup. With advanced post-processing techniques such as multi-plane

http://dx.doi.org/10.5772/56021

reconstruction, I-slice and excellent temporal resolution of narrow-sector acquisition with the anatomical definition of wide-sector acquisition, the multi-disciplinary TAVR team is now able to perform this important procedure with great precision and with minimal risk.

Author details

Daniel Zalkind, Michael Kim and Ernesto E. Salcedo

*Address all correspondence to: ernesto.e.salcedo@ucdenver.edu

University of Colorado Hospital Anschutz Medical Campus, USA

References

[1] Leon, M. B, Smith, C. R, Mack, M, et al. Transcatheter aortic-valve implantation for aortic stenosis in patients who cannot undergo surgery. N Engl J Med (2010). , 363, 1597-607.

[2] Baumgartner, H, Hung, J, Bermejo, J, et al. Echocardiographic assessment of valve stenosis: EAE/ASE recommendations for clinical practice. J Am Soc Echocardiogr (2009). quiz 101-2., 22, 1-23.

[3] Blanke, P, Euringer, W, Baumann, T, et al. Combined assessment of aortic root anatomy and aortoiliac vasculature with dual-source CT as a screening tool in patients evaluated for ranscatheter aortic valve implantation. Am J Roentgenol (2010). , 195, 872-81.

[4] Blanke, P, Siepe, M, Reinohl, J, et al. Assessment of aortic annulus dimensions for Edwards SAPIEN Transapical Heart Valve implantation by computed tomography: calculating average diameter using a virtual ring method. Eur J Cardiothorac Surg (2010). , 38, 750-8.

[5] Delgado, V, Ng, A. C, Schuijf, J. D, et al. Automated assessment of the aortic root dimensions with multidetector row computed tomography. Ann Thorac Surg (2011). , 91, 716-23.

[6] Kurra, V, Kapadia, S. R, Tuzcu, E. M, et al. Pre-procedural imaging of aortic root orientation and dimensions: comparison between X-ray angiographic planar imaging and 3-dimensional multidetector row computed tomography. JACC Cardiovasc Interv (2010). , 3, 105-13.

[7] Bagur, R, Rodes-cabau, J, Doyle, D, et al. Usefulness of TEE as the primary imaging echnique to guide transcatheter transapical aortic valve implantation. JACC Cardiovasc maging (2011). , 4, 115-24.

[8] Anderson, R. H. Clinical anatomy of the aortic root. Heart (2000). , 84, 670-3.

[9] Ho, S. Y. Structure and anatomy of the aortic root. Eur J Echocardiogr (2009). i , 3-10.

[10] Piazza, N, De Jaegere, P, Schultz, C, Becker, A. E, Serruys, P. W, & Anderson, R. H. Anatomy of the aortic valvar complex and its implications for transcatheter implantation of the aortic valve. Circ Cardiovasc Interv (2008). , 1, 74-81.

[11] Dashkevich, A, Blanke, P, Siepe, M, et al. Preoperative assessment of aortic annulus dimensions: comparison of noninvasive and intraoperative measurement. Ann Thorac Surg (2011). , 91, 709-14.

[12] Devereux, R. B, Alonso, D. R, & Lutas, E. M. et. al. Echocardiographic assessment of left ventricular hypertrophy: comparison to necropsy findings. American Journal of Cardiology (1986). , 57, 450-8.

[13] Ibid. Baumgartner

[14] Veronesi, F, Corsi, C, Sugeng, L, et al. A study of functional anatomy of aortic-mitral valve coupling using 3D matrix transesophageal echocardiography. Circ Cardiovasc Imaging (2009). , 2, 24-31.

[15] Tseng, W, Meineri, M, & Hahn, R. et. Al. Effect of transcatheter aortic valve replacement on the mitral valve. Moderated Poster Contribution. JACC (2012). s1): E , 1260-1260.

[16] Martin, A. G, Ruiz, J. M, & Gonzalez, A. E. et. al. Multiplane Transesophageal Echocardiography in the Preoperative Evaluation of the Sinus of Valsalva Fistula to Right Chambers. Rev Esp Cardiol. (2002).

[17] Shanewise, J. S, Cheung, A. T, & Aronson, S. et. al. ASE/SCA Guidelines for Performing a Comprehensive Intraoperative Multiplant Transesophageal Echocardiography Examination. JASE (1999). , 12, 884-900.

[18] Beraud, A. S, Schnittger, I, & Miller, D. C. et. al. Multiplanar reconstruction of three-dimensional transthoracic echocardiography improves the presurgical assessment of mitral prolapse. JASE (2009).

[19] Sutton, J. P. rd, Ho SY, Anderson RH. The forgotten interleaflet triangles: a review of the surgical anatomy of the aortic valve. Ann Thorac Surg (1995). , 59, 419-27.

[20] Roberts, W. C, Vowels, T. J, Ko, J. M, et al. Comparison of the structure of the aortic valve and ascending aorta in adults having aortic valve replacement for aortic stenosis versus for pure aortic regurgitation and resection of the ascending aorta for aneurysm. Circulation (2011). , 123, 896-903.

[21] Caselli, S, Mazzesi, G, Tritapepe, L, et al. D echocardiographic delineation of mitral-aortic ntervalular fibrosa pseudoaneurysm caused by bicuspid aortic valve endocarditis. Echocardiography (2011). E , 1-4.

[22] Frommelt, M. A, Snider, A. R, & Bove, E. L. et. al. Echocardiographic assessment of subvalvular aortic stenosis before and after operation. JACC (1992). , 19, 1018-1023.

[23] Nagueh, S. E, Bierig, S. M, & Budoff, M. J. et. al. American Society of Echocardiography Clinical Recommendations for Multimodality Cardiovascular Imaging of Patient with Hypertrophic Cardiomyopathy. JASE (2011). , 24, 473-98.

[24] Ibid. Bagur

[25] Shiotavon Ramm, et. al. Real-time Three-dimensional Echocardiography for Determining Right Ventricular Stroke Volume in an Animal Model of Chronic Right Ventricular Volume Overload. Circulation. (1998). , 97, 1897-1900.

[26] GopalKing, et. al. Left ventricular volume and endocardial surface area by three-dimensional echocardiography: comparison with two-dimensional echocardiography and nuclear magnetic resonance imaging in normal subjects. JACC(1993).

[27] Araiet. al. Accuracy of measurement LVEF by new real-time three-dimensional echocardiography…AJC(2004).

[28] Langet. al. Three-Dimensional Echocardiography: The Benefits of the Additional Dimension. JACC (2006).

[29] Goland, S, & Trento, A. Iida Kiyoshi, et. al. Assessment of aortic stenosis by three-dimensional echocardiography: an accurate and novel approach. Heart (2007). , 93, 801-807.

[30] Monaghan, M. J. Role of real time 3D echocardiography in evaluating the left ventricle. Heart (2006).

[31] Adegunsoye, A, Mundkur, M, Nanda, N. C, & Hage, F. G. Echocardiographic evaluation of calcific aortic stenosis in the older adult. Echocardiography (2011). , 28, 117-29.

[32] Baumgartner, H, Hung, J, & Bermejo, J. et. al. Echocardiographic assessment of valve stenosis: EAE/ASE recommendations for clinical practice. European Journal of Echocardiography (2009). , 10, 1-25.

[33] Carabello, B. A, & Paulus, W. J. Aortic stenosis. Lancet (2009). , 373, 956-66.

[34] Ng, A. C, Delgado, V, & Van Der Kley, F. et. al. Comparison of aortic root dimensions and geometries before and after transcatheter aortic valve implantation by 2- and 3- dimensional tranesophageal echocardiography and multislice computed tomography. Circulation Cardiovascular Imaging (2010). , 3, 94-102.

[35] Ozkan, M, Gunduz, S, & Yildiz, M. et. al. Diagnosis of the prosthetic heart valve pannus formation with real-time three-dimensional transoesophageal echocardiography. European Journal of Echocardiography (2010). E17

[36] Clavel, M-A, Rodes-cabau, J, & Dumont, E. et. al. Validation and characterization of transcatheter aortic valve effective orifice area measured by Doppler echocardiography. JACC Imaging (2011). , 4, 1053-62.

[37] Lancellotti, P, Tribouilloy, C, & Hagendorgg, A. et. al. EAE recommendations for the assessment of valvular regurgitation. Part I: aortic and pulmonary regurgitation. European Journal of Echocardiography (2010). , 11(3), 223-244.

[38] Karalis, D. G, Bansal, R. C, Hauck, A. J, et al. Transesophageal echocardiographic recognition of subaortic complications in aortic valve endocarditis. Clinical and surgical implications. Circulation (1992). , 86, 353-62.

[39] Simpson, I. A, De Belder, M. A, & Kenny, A. et. al. How to quantify valve regurgitation by echo Doppler techniques. British Heart Journal (1995). , 73, 1-9.

[40] Fang, L, Hsiung, M. C, & Miller, A. P. et. al. Assessment of aortic regurgitation by live three0dimensional transthoracic echocardiographic measurements of vena contracta area: usefulness and validation. Echocardiography (2005). , 22, 775-81.

[41] Pouleur, A-C. le Polain de Waroux J-B, et. al. Accuracy of the flow convergence method for quantification of aortic regurgitation in patients with central versus eccentric jets. American Journal of Cardiology (2008). , 102, 475-80.

[42] Pate, G, & Thomson, C. R. Munt Bl, et. al. Techniques for percutaneous closure of prosthetic paravalvular leaks. Catheter Cardiovascular Interventions. (2010). , 67, 158-66.

[43] Koos, R, Mahnken, A. H, & Dohmen, G. et. al. Association of aortic valve calcification severity with the degree of aortic regurgitation after transcatheter aortic valve implantation. Int J Cardiol (2010). , 150, 142-5.

[44] Schultz, C, Rossi, A, Van Mieghem, N, & Van Der Boon, R. et. al. Aortic annulus dimensions and leaflet calcification from contrast MSCT predict the need for balloon post-dilatation after TAVI with the Medtronic CoreValve prosthesis. Eurointevention, (2011). , 2011(7), 5-564.

[45] Sherif, M. A, Abdel-wahab, M, & Stocker, B. et. al. Anatomic and procedural predictors of paravalvular aortic regurgitation after implantation of the Medtronic CoreValve bioprosthesis. JACC (2010). , 56, 1623-9.

[46] Kodali, S. K, Williams, M. R, & Smith, C. R. Et. al. Two-Year Outcomes after Transcatheter or Surgical Aortic-Valve Replacement. NEJM. 366; , 18, 1686-1695.

[47] Ibid. Bagur

[48] Dashkevich, A, Blanke, P, Siepe, M, et al. Preoperative assessment of aortic annulus dimensions: comparison of noninvasive and intraoperative measurement. Ann Thorac Surg (2011). , 91, 709-14.

[49] Rodes-cabau, J, Dumont, E, Boone, R. H, et al. Cerebral embolism following transcatheter aortic valve implantation: comparison of transfemoral and transapical approaches. J Am Coll Cardiol (2011). , 57, 18-28.

[50] Tzikas, A, Geleijnse, M. L, Van Mieghem, N. M, et al. Left ventricular mass regression one year after transcatheter aortic valve implantation. Ann Thorac Surg (2011). , 91, 685-91.

[51] Lerakis, S, Babaliaros, V. C, & Block, P. C. et. al. Transesophageal echocardiography to help position and deploy a transcatheter heart valve. JACC Imaging (2010). , 3, 219-21.

[52] Filgueiras-rama, D, Lopez, T, & Moreno-gomez, R. et. al. 3D transesophageal echocardiographic guidance and monitoring of percutaneous aortic valve replacement. Echocardiography (2010). , 27, 84-6.

[53] Jayasuriya, C, Moss, R. R, & Munr, B. Transcatheter Aortic Valve Implantation in Aortic Stenosis: The Role of Echocardiography. JASE. (2011). , 24(1), 15-27.

[54] Durand, E, Borz, B, & Godin, M. et. al. Transfemoral aortic valve replacement with the Edwards SAPIEN and Edwards SAPIEN XT prosthesis using exclusively local anesthesia and fluoroscopic guidance: feasibility and 30-day outcomes. JACC Cardiovascular Interventions. (2012). May; , 5(5), 461-7.

[55] Schultz, C. J, Tzikas, A, Moelker, A, & Rossi, A. et. al. Correlates on MSCT of paravalvular aortic regurgitation after aortic valve implantation using the Medtronic COreValve prosthesis. Catheter Cardiovasc Interv, (2011). , 2011(78), 3-446.

[56] Ibid Jayasuriya

[57] Shames, S, Koczo, A, & Hahn, R. et. al. In-stent flow acceleration in the SAPIEN trans-catheter aortic valve: impact on the echocardiographic assessment of valve function. JASE (2011).

[58] IbidBlanke, Delgado, Kurra

[59] Schultz, C. J, Molker, A, & Piazza, N. et. al. Three dimensional evaluation of the aortic annulus using multislice computer tomography. European Heart Journal (2010). , 31, 849-856.

[60] Gurvitch, R, Webb, J, & Yuan, R. et. al. Aortic annulus diameter determination by multidetector computed tomography: reproducibility, applicability and implications for transcatheter aortic valve implantation. JACC Intervention. (2011). , 4, 1235-45.

[61] Bloomfield, G. S, Gillam, L. D, & Hahn, R. T. et. al. A Practical guide to multimodality imaging of transcatheter aortic valve replacement. JACC Imaging (2012). , 5, 441-455.

[62] Jilaihawi, H, Kashif, M, & Fontana, G. et. al. Cross-Sectional Computed Tomographic Assessment Improves Accuracy of Aortic Annular Sizing for Transcatheter Aortic

Valve Replacement and Reduces the Incidence of Paravalvular Aortic Regurgitation. JACC(2012).

[63] Ibid. Tadros.

[64] Burgstahler, C, Kunze, M, & Loeflller, C. et. al. Assessment of left ventricular outflow tract geometry in non-stenotic and stenotic aortic valves by cardiovascular magnetic resonance.Journal of Cardiovascular Magnetic Resonance (2006). , 8, 825-9.

[65] Lee, A. P, Lam, Y. Y, Yip, G. W, & Lang, R. M. et. al. Role of real time three-dimensional transesophageal echocardiography in guidance of interventional proedures in cardiology. Heart (2010). , 96, 1485-1493.